State-of-the-Art in Orthodontics and Gnathology

State-of-the-Art in Orthodontics and Gnathology

Editors

Giuseppe Minervini
Fabrizia d'Apuzzo
Vincenzo Grassia

MDPI • Basel • Beijing • Wuhan • Barcelona • Belgrade • Manchester • Tokyo • Cluj • Tianjin

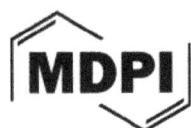

Editors
Giuseppe Minervini
University of Campania Luigi Vanvitelli
Italy

Fabrizia d'Apuzzo
University of Campania Luigi Vanvitelli
Italy

Vincenzo Grassia
University of Campania Luigi Vanvitelli
Italy

Editorial Office
MDPI
St. Alban-Anlage 66
4052 Basel, Switzerland

This is a reprint of articles from the Special Issue published online in the open access journal *Applied Sciences* (ISSN 2076-3417) (available at: https://www.mdpi.com/journal/applsci/special_issues/Orthodontics_Gnathology).

For citation purposes, cite each article independently as indicated on the article page online and as indicated below:

LastName, A.A.; LastName, B.B.; LastName, C.C. Article Title. *Journal Name* **Year**, *Volume Number*, Page Range.

ISBN 978-3-0365-6936-9 (Hbk)
ISBN 978-3-0365-6937-6 (PDF)

© 2023 by the authors. Articles in this book are Open Access and distributed under the Creative Commons Attribution (CC BY) license, which allows users to download, copy and build upon published articles, as long as the author and publisher are properly credited, which ensures maximum dissemination and a wider impact of our publications.

The book as a whole is distributed by MDPI under the terms and conditions of the Creative Commons license CC BY-NC-ND.

Contents

About the Editors vii

Preface to "State-of-the-Art in Orthodontics and Gnathology" ix

Giuseppe Minervini
State-of-the-Art in Orthodontics and Gnathology
Reprinted from: *Appl. Sci.* **2022**, *12*, 12419, doi:10.3390/app122312419 1

Matthew Gibson, Randy Q. Cron, Matthew L. Stoll, Brian E. Kinard, Tessa Patterson and Chung How Kau
A 3D CBCT Analysis of Airway and Cephalometric Values in Patients Diagnosed with Juvenile Idiopathic Arthritis Compared to a Control Group
Reprinted from: *Appl. Sci.* **2022**, *12*, 4286, doi:10.3390/app12094286 5

Jovana Juloski, Dina Vasovic, Ljiljana Vucic, Tina Pajevic, Nevena Gligoric, Mladen Mirkovic and Branislav Glisic
Predictors of Analgesic Consumption in Orthodontic Patients
Reprinted from: *Appl. Sci.* **2022**, *12*, 3390, doi:10.3390/app12073390 19

Livia Nastri, Ludovica Nucci, Domenico Carozza, Stefano Martina, Ismene Serino, Letizia Perillo, et al.
Gingival Recessions and Periodontal Status after Minimum 2-Year-Retention Post-Non-Extraction Orthodontic Treatment
Reprinted from: *Appl. Sci.* **2022**, *12*, 1641, doi:10.3390/app12031641 27

Fabrizia d'Apuzzo, Ludovica Nucci, Bruno M. Strangio, Alessio Danilo Inchingolo, Gianna Dipalma, Giuseppe Minervini, et al.
Dento-Skeletal Class III Treatment with Mixed Anchored Palatal Expander: A Systematic Review
Reprinted from: *Appl. Sci.* **2022**, *12*, 4646, doi:10.3390/app12094646 37

Giuseppina Malcangi, Alessio Danilo Inchingolo, Assunta Patano, Giovanni Coloccia, Sabino Ceci, Mariagrazia Garibaldi, et al.
Impacted Central Incisors in the Upper Jaw in an Adolescent Patient: Orthodontic-Surgical Treatment—A Case Report
Reprinted from: *Appl. Sci.* **2022**, *12*, 2657, doi:10.3390/app12052657 53

About the Editors

Giuseppe Minervini

Dr. Giuseppe Minervini graduated in Dental Medicine in July 2016 with honors. During his undergraduate course, he attended the "Rey Juan Carlos Alcorcon" in Madrid (Spain) between September 2013 and June 2014 for the Erasmus project. He received his Postgraduate Diploma in Orthodontics in December 2020 from the University of Campania Luigi Vanvitelli, Naples, Italy. Dr. Minervini is currently a PhD student in Biochemistry and Biotechnology at the University of Campania Luigi Vanvitelli, Naples, Italy. He was a visiting scholar as part of the Tweed Study Course in 2019 at Charles H. Tweed International Foundation, Tucson, Arizona. He is Subject Expert in Dental Materials and a tutor in the Orthodontics Dentistry School at the University of Campania Luigi Vanvitelli, Naples, Italy. He is also Executive Guest Editor for several Special Issues and a member of the SIDO, EOS. Dr. Minervini has published several articles and posters (h-index: 18) as author or co-author. He has received several awards and distinctions. His research interests include biomedical and biomaterials application for the craniofacial, oral, and temporomandibular area, dentofacial orthopedics, orofacial pain, temporomandibular joint disorders, prothesis, oral pathology, orthodontics, and teledentistry.

Fabrizia d'Apuzzo

Dr. Fabrizia d'Apuzzo graduated in Dentistry in 2012, subsequently obtaining her master's degree in Orthodontics, in 2017, and Doctorate in Biochemical and Biotechnological Sciences in 2019 at the University of Campania Luigi Vanvitelli in Naples (Italy). As part of her study and/or research duties during her education, she attended the University of Lille II (French), University of Trieste (Italy), and Virginia Commonwealth University in Richmond, VA (USA). She is currently a Postdoctoral Research Fellow at the Multidisciplinary Department of Medical-Surgical and Dental Specialties, a position she has served since 2019, and a Subject Expert in Orthodontics and Orofacial Pain in the Dental Hygiene course, both at the University of Campania Luigi Vanvitelli in Naples (Italy).

Vincenzo Grassia

Prof. Vincenzo Grassia graduated in Dental Medicine in 2007 with honors. He received his Postgraduate Diploma in Orthodontics in 2011 at the Second University of Naples and completed his orthodontic training with a PhD in Chemical, Biological, and Biotechnological Sciences at the Second University of Naples in 2016. He is currently Assistant Professor at the University of Campania Luigi Vanvitelli. He is certificated by the IBO (Italian Board of Orthodontics), EBO (European Board of Orthodontics), and IBOA (Italian Board of Orthodontic Aligner) in addition to being a member of the SIDO, EOS, WFO, and SIALIGN. Dr. Grassia is author and co-author of more than 40 publications, 3 book chapters, and over 40 posters. He has been a speaker at national and international conferences, where he has received numerous awards and distinctions. His research interests include tooth movements, dentofacial orthopedics, and orthodontic biomechanism, digital orthodontics, clear aligners, mini-screws, and early treatment.

Preface to "State-of-the-Art in Orthodontics and Gnathology"

The objective of this book is to present the main evidence-based data on new developments and knowledge in diagnostic and treatment technologies in the orofacial field used in both children and adults. The published content has been met with great success in interdisciplinary fields, stimulating international authors to submit their original articles, reviews, or case reports based on various aspects of orthodontics as well as on the diagnosis and management of temporomandibular disorders and orofacial pain. Among the current highly debated topics, this Book focuses on multiple disciplines as follows: gingival recessions and periodontal status after orthodontic treatment; a rare case of impacted central incisors; predictors of analgesic consumption in orthodontic patients; a systematic review about different dentoskeletal class III treatment approaches; evaluation of upper airway volumes; and cephalometric values in JIA patients.

Giuseppe Minervini, Fabrizia d'Apuzzo, and Vincenzo Grassia
Editors

Editorial

State-of-the-Art in Orthodontics and Gnathology

Giuseppe Minervini

Multidisciplinary Department of Medical-Surgical and Dental Specialties, University of Campania Luigi Vanvitelli, via Luigi De Crecchio 6, 80138 Naples, Italy; giuseppe.minervini@unicampania.it; Tel.: +39-3289129558

Citation: Minervini, G. State-of-the-Art in Orthodontics and Gnathology. *Appl. Sci.* **2022**, *12*, 12419. https://doi.org/10.3390/app122312419

Received: 19 November 2022
Accepted: 24 November 2022
Published: 5 December 2022

Publisher's Note: MDPI stays neutral with regard to jurisdictional claims in published maps and institutional affiliations.

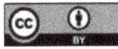

Copyright: © 2022 by the author. Licensee MDPI, Basel, Switzerland. This article is an open access article distributed under the terms and conditions of the Creative Commons Attribution (CC BY) license (https://creativecommons.org/licenses/by/4.0/).

In recent years, several novel diagnostic and treatment modalities have been introduced in orthodontics and temporomandibular disorders [1,2]. Researchers and clinicians are called to update themselves according to the developments occurring in these fields. New technologies and digital devices are able to accelerate the diagnostic process and increase the effectiveness in diagnosing dysfunctions in the orofacial region [3]. Furthermore, thanks to intraoral scanners, digital dental and skeletal models, facial scanning, cone beam computed tomography (CBCT), magnetic resonance imaging (MRI), digital smile design (DSD), photogrammetry, and artificial intelligence (AI), diagnoses are becoming increasingly accurate, particularly in complex cases with impacted teeth, dental transpositions, and orofacial disharmonies and anomalies [2]. In addition, patients are becoming increasingly demanding regarding treatment time and aesthetics [4]; thus, different methods such as corticotomy, pulsed light, mechanical vibrations to accelerate orthodontic movement, or an increase in the use of clear brackets and aligners are more common than in previous decades [5–7]. The objective of this Special Issue was to present the main evidence-based data on new developments and knowledge in diagnostic and treatment technologies in the orofacial field used in both children and adults. The articles published in this Collection have been met with great success in interdisciplinary fields, stimulating international authors to submit their original articles, reviews, or case reports based on various aspects of orthodontics, as well as on the diagnosis and management of temporomandibular disorders and orofacial pain [8–12]. Among the current highly debated topics, this Special Issue focused on multiple disciplines as follows: gingival recessions and periodontal status after orthodontic treatment; a rare case of impacted central incisors; predictors of analgesic consumption in orthodontic patients; a systematic review about different dento-skeletal class III treatment approaches; upper airway volumes evaluation, cephalometric values in JIA patients [8–12].

Specifically, the manuscript titled "Dento-Skeletal Class III Treatment with Mixed Anchored Palatal Expander: A Systematic Review" [8] aimed to determine the efficacy of using a mixed anchored palatal expander to treat Class III malocclusions, as well as to observe whether using a bone-anchorage device induces more maxillary advancement with fewer dental side effects. These treatment approaches are among the most currently used in the treatment of moderate-to-severe Class III malocclusions. This review was well conducted by following the more recent PROSPERO guidelines redacted for the International Prospective Register of Systematic Reviews (Centre for Reviews and Dissemination, University of York, York, UK). The authors concluded that combining tooth-borne and bone-borne appliances for rapid maxillary extension may be advised in treatment protocols for skeletal Class III patients to obtain more skeletal results while lowering maxillary dentition side effects [8].

Another publication of Nastri et al. [11] aimed to assess the gingival recessions (GR) and periodontal status in a group of young patients previously treated with non-extraction orthodontic treatments and retention, with a minimum two-year follow up after the end of active treatment. In particular, they selected data from patients with a previous non-extractive orthodontic treatment, and at least two years of storage and complete records were collected before and after treatment. Dental models were digitized with the 3Shape TRIOS® intraoral scanner, a new technology, and Viewbox4 software was used for the measurements. The following parameters were considered: inclination of the lower and upper incisors (IMPA and I^SN) and anterior crowding (Little index). The follow-up periodontal clinical examination considered the following parameters: buccal and lingual GR (mm) of incisors and canines, probing score bleeding, plaque score and phenotype gingival. At the follow-up periodontal visits, patients had low overall oral hygiene with bleeding at probing in 66.6% and plaque in the anterior area in 76.2% of patients. From the total examined 240 teeth of the frontal sextants, only three patients showed GR, and the gingival phenotype was thick in 55% of cases. Based on the results, the non-extractive orthodontic treatment would appear not to affect the development of buccal or lingual recessions or the periodontal state after at least two years of post-orthodontic retention. A slight increase in the risk of developing buccal RBC was detected only in correlation with the presence of a fixed retainer and thin gingival phenotype, mainly in patients with gingivitis. Thus, this research will be extremely useful for clinicians in order to schedule periodical periodontal follow-up appointments, mainly in patients after orthodontic treatment, in order to motivate them to maintain better oral hygiene in adulthood [11].

The paper of Malcangi et al. [9] described a rare case of orthodontic-surgical treatment. In particular, they described a case of inclusion of both maxillary permanent central incisors. This situation negatively affects facial appearance, phonation, and mastication function. As a consequence, early diagnosis is essential to avoid complications and failures. Various reasons for the inclusion were identified, but supernumerary teeth were the leading cause. Early causes of removal and the rapid expansion of the palate show a great chance of success with the spontaneous eruption of the impacted elements; however, surgical orthodontic treatment is often necessary. The inclination of the teeth with respect to the midline and the root maturation degree establishes prognosis and therapeutic times. In this clinical case, a 9-year-old boy showed two impacted supernumerary teeth in the anterior maxillary region, hindering the eruption of the permanent upper central incisors. The impacted supernumerary teeth were surgically removed at different times. A straight wire multibracket technique associated with a fixed palatal appliance was chosen. The palatal appliance consisted of an osteomucosal resin support at the level of the retroincisal papilla. Subsequently, surgical exposure was performed using the closed eruption and elastic traction technique, bringing 11 and 21 back into the arch. The authors concluded that an early and accurate diagnosis supported by clinical and radiological examinations, such as OPG X-ray and CBCT, is crucial. It is essential to evaluate the predictive eruption factor that conditions the treatment plan, such as: patient age, history, compliance, distance from the occlusal plane, vertical position of non-erupted incisors, and inclination with respect to the midline. Complication during tooth eruption could negatively affect the occlusion development and the child's psychology. The early orthodontic interceptive treatment with the elimination of the obstacle and orthopedic expansion with RME is fundamental. In general, the surgical-orthodontic treatment of impacted incisors has a good chance of success, but it takes time. It is essential to inform patients and their parents of the risk of failure and increase in treatment times, especially when the impacted incisors are in a very high alveolar position [9].

With their paper "Predictors of Analgesic Consumption in Orthodontic Patients", Juloski et al. [12] analyzed the predictors of analgesics consumption and identified the predictive factors for the self-administration of analgesics in orthodontic patients after the initiation of treatment with multibracket fixed appliances. During orthodontic treatment, pain is a subjective experience influenced by several factors, and patients use analgesics at different rates to relieve this pain without any specific guideline. Thus, the correlations between orthodontic pain and analgesic consumption were investigated after the beginning of orthodontic treatment with fixed appliances, in order to predict them. In a diary, for seven days, the 286 patients who participated in this study recorded their pain intensity (using a 0–10 numerical rating scale), analgesic usage, pain localization, pain triggers, and pain characteristics. Univariable analyses revealed the presence of potential predictive factors: age, gender, pain intensity, pain localization, pain while chewing, pain at rest, night pain, headache, pulsating pain, sharp pain, dull pain, and tingling. Multivariate analyses revealed that increasing age, increasing pain intensity, and the presence of a headache all increased analgesic consumption. Overall, the model explained 33% of the variability in analgesic requirement. Analgesic use has been shown to be predicted by age, pain intensity, and headache, and knowledge of these factors can facilitate clinicians in identifying orthodontic patients who will consume analgesics on their own. In the conclusion, the authors affirmed that age, intensity of pain, and headache are fair predictors for analgesic consumption [12].

The last paper, by Gibson et al. [10], evaluated the upper airway volumes and cephalometric values in juvenile idiopathic arthritis (JIA) patients compared to healthy controls. The temporomandibular joint (TMJ) is involved in 30–45% of patients with all JIA subtypes. These subjects may show altered craniofacial morphology such as micrognathia, retrognathia, hyperdivergent mandibular plane angle, and skeletal anterior open bite. These features are also associated with non-JIA pediatric patients with obstructive sleep apnea (OSA). The research included a group of 32 JIA patients and a group of 32 healthy subjects. A CBCT was requested from each patient, and the DICOM files were imported into Dolphin Imaging software to measure the upper airway volumes and the most constricted cross-sectional areas of each patient. The cephalometric images were exported from the CBCT data for each patient, and several cephalometric values were assessed. All measurements were compared between the JIA and control groups. For airway values, statistically significant differences were found in the nasopharynx airway volume, total upper airway volume, and the most constricted cross-sectional area, whereas the oropharyngeal airway volume did not show significance. In the cephalometrics, a statistically significant difference was found for the posterior facial height.

In conclusion, this study showed that there was a difference in the posterior face height, as well as a significant difference in total upper airway volume, nasopharynx airway volume, and most constricted cross-sectional area measurements between the JIA and control patients.

Specifically, 50% of JIA patients had an airway with a most constricted cross-sectional area of less than 100 mm^2, and 67% had an asymmetric airway form [10].

Thus, this Special Issue will be helpful in evaluating the most current and significant interdisciplinary diagnostic and treatment approaches currently available in orthodontics and TMD management in both young and adult patients.

Funding: This research received no external funding.

Institutional Review Board Statement: Not applicable.

Informed Consent Statement: Not applicable.

Conflicts of Interest: The authors declare no conflict of interest.

References

1. Scribante, A.; Gallo, S.; Bertino, K.; Meles, S.; Gandini, P.; Sfondrini, M.F. The Effect of Chairside Verbal Instructions Matched with Instagram Social Media on Oral Hygiene of Young Orthodontic Patients: A Randomized Clinical Trial. *Appl. Sci.* **2021**, *11*, 706. [CrossRef]
2. Pasciuti, E.; Coloccia, G.; Inchingolo, A.D.; Patano, A.; Ceci, S.; Bordea, I.R.; Cardarelli, F.; Di Venere, D.; Inchingolo, F.; Dipalma, G. Deep Bite Treatment with Aligners: A New Protocol. *Appl. Sci.* **2022**, *12*, 6709. [CrossRef]
3. Sfondrini, M.; Butera, A.; Di Michele, P.; Luccisano, C.; Ottini, B.; Sangalli, E.; Gallo, S.; Pascadopoli, M.; Gandini, P.; Scribante, A. Microbiological Changes during Orthodontic Aligner Therapy: A Prospective Clinical Trial. *Appl. Sci.* **2021**, *11*, 6758. [CrossRef]
4. Scrascia, R.; Cicciù, M.; Manco, C.; Miccoli, A.; Cervino, G. Angled Screwdriver Solutions and Low-Profile Attachments in Full Arch Rehabilitation with Divergent Implants. *Appl. Sci.* **2021**, *11*, 1122. [CrossRef]
5. Sfondrini, M.F.; Pascadopoli, M.; Dicorato, S.; Todaro, C.; Nardi, M.G.; Gallo, S.; Gandini, P.; Scribante, A. Bone Modifications Induced by Rapid Maxillary Expander: A Three-Dimensional Cephalometric Pilot Study Comparing Two Different Cephalometric Software Programs. *Appl. Sci.* **2022**, *12*, 4313. [CrossRef]

6. Inchingolo, A.D.; Carpentiere, V.; Piras, F.; Netti, A.; Ferrara, I.; Campanelli, M.; Latini, G.; Viapiano, F.; Costa, S.; Malcangi, G.; et al. Orthodontic Surgical Treatment of Impacted Mandibular Canines: Systematic Review and Case Report. *Appl. Sci.* **2022**, *12*, 8008. [CrossRef]
7. Scribante, A.; Gallo, S.; Pascadopoli, M.; Canzi, P.; Marconi, S.; Montasser, M.A.; Bressani, D.; Gandini, P.; Sfondrini, M.F. Properties of CAD/CAM 3D Printing Dental Materials and Their Clinical Applications in Orthodontics: Where Are We Now? *Appl. Sci.* **2022**, *12*, 551. [CrossRef]
8. D'Apuzzo, F.; Nucci, L.; Strangio, B.M.; Inchingolo, A.D.; Dipalma, G.; Minervini, G.; Perillo, L.; Grassia, V. Dento-Skeletal Class III Treatment with Mixed Anchored Palatal Expander: A Systematic Review. *Appl. Sci.* **2022**, *12*, 4646. [CrossRef]
9. Malcangi, G.; Inchingolo, A.D.; Patano, A.; Coloccia, G.; Ceci, S.; Garibaldi, M.; Inchingolo, A.M.; Piras, F.; Cardarelli, F.; Settanni, V.; et al. Impacted Central Incisors in the Upper Jaw in an Adolescent Patient: Orthodontic-Surgical Treatment—A Case Report. *Appl. Sci.* **2022**, *12*, 2657. [CrossRef]
10. Gibson, M.; Cron, R.Q.; Stoll, M.L.; Kinard, B.E.; Patterson, T.; Kau, C.H. A 3D CBCT Analysis of Airway and Cephalometric Values in Patients Diagnosed with Juvenile Idiopathic Arthritis Compared to a Control Group. *Appl. Sci.* **2022**, *12*, 4286. [CrossRef]
11. Nastri, L.; Nucci, L.; Carozza, D.; Martina, S.; Serino, I.; Perillo, L.; D'Apuzzo, F.; Grassia, V. Gingival Recessions and Periodontal Status after Minimum 2-Year-Retention Post-Non-Extraction Orthodontic Treatment. *Appl. Sci.* **2022**, *12*, 1641. [CrossRef]
12. Juloski, J.; Vasovic, D.; Vucic, L.; Pajevic, T.; Gligoric, N.; Mirkovic, M.; Glisic, B. Predictors of Analgesic Consumption in Orthodontic Patients. *Appl. Sci.* **2022**, *12*, 3390. [CrossRef]

Short Biography of Author

Dr. Giuseppe Minervini graduated in Dental Medicine in July 2016 with honors. During his undergraduate course, he attended the "Rey Juan Carlos Alcorcon" in Madrid (Spain) between September 2013 and June 2014 for the Erasmus project. He received his Postgraduate Diploma in Orthodontics in December 2020 from the University of Campania, Luigi Vanvitelli, Naples, Italy. Dr. Minervini is currently a PhD student in Biochemistry and Biotechnology at the University of Campania, Luigi Vanvitelli, Naples, Italy. He visited the scholar Tweed Study Course in 2019 at Charles H. Tweed International Foundation, Tucson, Arizona. He is Subject Expert in Dental Materials and a tutor in the Orthodontics Dentistry School at the University of Campania Luigi Vanvitelli, Naples, Italy. He is also Executive Guest Editor for several Special Issues and a member of the SIDO, EOS. Dr. Minervini has published several articles and posters (h-index: 12) as an author or co-author. He has received several awards and distinctions. His research interests include biomedical and biomaterials application for the craniofacial, oral and temporomandibular area, dentofacial orthopedics, orofacial pain, temporomandibular joint disorders, prothesis, oral pathology, orthodontics, and teledentistry.

Article

A 3D CBCT Analysis of Airway and Cephalometric Values in Patients Diagnosed with Juvenile Idiopathic Arthritis Compared to a Control Group

Matthew Gibson [1], Randy Q. Cron [2], Matthew L. Stoll [2], Brian E. Kinard [3], Tessa Patterson [1] and Chung How Kau [1,*]

1. Department of Orthodontics, University of Alabama at Birmingham, Birmingham, AL 35294, USA; mg308@uab.edu (M.G.); tep1101@uab.edu (T.P.)
2. Department of Pediatric Rheumatology, University of Alabama at Birmingham, Birmingham, AL 35233, USA; randycron@uabmc.edu (R.Q.C.); mstoll@uabmc.edu (M.L.S.)
3. Department of Oral and Maxillofacial Surgery, University of Alabama at Birmingham, Birmingham, AL 35294, USA; briankinard@uabmc.edu
* Correspondence: ckau@uab.edu

Abstract: Introduction: The temporomandibular joint (TMJ) is affected in 30–45% of juvenile idiopathic arthritis (JIA) patients, with all JIA subtypes at risk for TMJ involvement. JIA patients with TMJ involvement may present with altered craniofacial morphology, including micrognathia, mandibular retrognathia, a hyperdivergent mandibular plane angle, and skeletal anterior open bite. These features are also commonly present and associated with non-JIA pediatric patients with obstructive sleep apnea (OSA). Materials and Methods: The study was comprised of a group of 32 JIA patients and a group of 32 healthy control subjects. CBCT images were taken for all patients and were imported into Dolphin Imaging software. The Dolphin Imaging was used to measure the upper airway volumes and the most constricted cross-sectional areas of each patient. Cephalometric images were rendered from the CBCT data for each patient, and the following cephalometric values were identified: SNA angle, SNB angle, ANB angle, anterior facial height (AFH), posterior facial height (PFH), mandibular plane angle (SN-MP), FMA (FH-MP), overjet (OJ), and overbite (OB). Airway volumes, the most constricted cross-sectional area values, and cephalometric values were compared between the JIA and control groups. Results: For airway values, statistically significant differences were seen in the nasopharynx airway volume ($p = 0.004$), total upper airway volume ($p = 0.013$), and the most constricted cross-sectional area ($p = 0.026$). The oropharynx airway volume was not statistically significant ($p = 0.051$). For cephalometric values, only the posterior facial height showed a statistically significant difference ($p = 0.024$). Conclusions: There was a significant difference in airway dimensions in the JIA patients as compared to the control patients. In addition, the posterior facial dimensions seem to be affected in JIA patients. The ODDs ratio analysis further corroborated the findings that were significant.

Keywords: 3D airway analysis; 3D airway volumes; CBCT; orthodontics; oral and maxillofacial surgery

1. Introduction

Juvenile idiopathic arthritis (JIA) is characterized by the onset of arthritis of an unknown etiology before the age of 16 that persists for longer than a six-week duration. JIA is the most common rheumatic disease of childhood [1–3]. The progression and course of disease in JIA is unpredictable. It is self-limiting in some patients while in other circumstances it can be persistent with joint resorption. Depending on the timing of onset and severity of disease, JIA may cause growth disturbances, permanent joint damage, functional limitations, and short- or long-term disability [4].

The temporomandibular joint (TMJ) is one of the more frequently involved synovial joints in JIA patients and in some cases may be the only joint involved [5,6]. The TMJ is affected in 30–45% of JIA patients, with all JIA subtypes at risk for TMJ involvement [7,8]. Despite the high percentage of JIA patients that have TMJ arthritis and a high prevalence of associated morbidity, TMJ arthritis is an underdiagnosed component of JIA [9]. This is due in part to the challenges associated with traditional radiography and clinical examination of the TMJ, as well as the fact that TMJ symptoms are frequently absent or unreliable [9–12]. Even with radiographic evidence of condylar lesions, a significant percentage of JIA patients do not report any TMJ symptoms and may have a benign clinical TMJ examination [5,13,14]. Despite these challenges, early diagnosis and treatment of TMJ arthritis is critical, as the risk of craniofacial growth alterations is thought to increase in cases of earlier age of onset and results in longer duration of disease activity [9,15].

As TMJ involvement may be present without any clinical signs or symptoms, MRI is the gold standard for diagnosis of TMJ involvement [14]. This imaging technique is capable of detecting 63–91% of inflammatory changes, ranging from active arthritic changes as well as the sequelae of chronic arthritis [10]. Higher percentages of TMJ involvement are found when Gadolinium-enhanced magnetic resonance imaging (Gd-MRI) is employed, compared to ultrasound, computed tomography (CT), cone-beam-computed tomography (CBCT), or traditional radiography (i.e., panoramic radiographs) [5,11,16–18].

The anatomy of the TMJ makes it particularly susceptible to damage from arthritis [5]. Unlike other synovial joints, the primary center for mandibular growth is the mandibular condylar cartilage that lies under a thin layer of fibrocartilage on the head of the condyle [5]. Due to its superficial position, it is susceptible to damage or resorption in the presence of chronic inflammation of the TMJ, and subsequently, TMJ arthritis may have destructive effects on the growth of the mandible [19,20]. JIA patients with TMJ involvement may present with altered craniofacial morphology, including micrognathia, mandibular retrognathism, decreased total mandibular length, decreased posterior face heights, increased anterior face heights, skeletal anterior open bite, posterior mandibular rotation with hyperdivergent mandibular plane angle and occlusal plane angle, obtuse gonial angle, gonial notching, convex facial profile, and facial asymmetry with chin deviation in cases of unilateral joint destruction [5,6,13,15,21–27]. In one study, retrognathia was seen in 82% of JIA patients that had TMJ involvement diagnosed using the panoramic radiograph but was also seen in 55% of patients that did not show any signs of radiographic TMJ involvement. Those patients who did have TMJ involvement had a cephalometric A point-nasion-B point (ANB) angle that averaged 1.8 degrees greater than those without TMJ involvement [6]. It has been shown that even a small degree of condylar damage can be associated with significant alterations in craniofacial morphology [13].

In recent years, CBCT has become a commonly used imaging modality in dentistry and orthodontics. Compared to traditional CT, CBCT has a shorter acquisition time and a more focused radiation beam with less scatter, resulting in lower radiation dosages and making it more appropriate for routine clinical use in a dental setting [28]. CBCT data can be used to assess skeletal craniofacial features and hard tissue structural abnormalities of the TMJ and can also provide a method of volumetric, cross-sectional area, and linear-dimensional airway analysis.

Several 3D airway studies have shown smaller airway volumes and the most constricted cross-sectional area (MCCA) measurements in adults with OSA, as measured by CBCT, but less research has been conducted on pediatric populations [29–33]. Recently, a study was undertaken to compare the apnea hypopnea index (AHI) measured by polysomnography (PSG) to CBCT measures in pediatric OSA patients, and it was concluded that CBCT analysis may be a useful tool in the evaluation of the upper airway in pediatric OSA patients [34]. It was shown in both the nasopharynx and oropharynx that airway volume as well as mean and minimal cross-sectional area were smaller in patients with moderate to severe OSA (AHI > 5) compared to primary snorers (AHI < 1) that were matched for age, gender, and obesity [34]. Another study relating AHI to CBCT airway data showed a statistically significant correlation between AHI and nasopharyngeal volume in children aged 7–11, as well as between AHI and the MCCA in the 12–17 age group [35].

Sleep-disordered breathing (SDB) and obstructive sleep apnea (OSA) may be among the functional impairments that JIA patients experience, which have been shown to be associated with pain, fatigue, and reduced health-related quality of life [36–38]. Daytime effects of OSA in children may include attention deficit, aggressive/impulsive behavior, hyperactivity, mood problems (including possibly depression/anxiety), poor school performance, headaches, fatigue, and excessive daytime sleepiness [39,40]. Although OSA is not caused by anatomic factors alone, certain craniofacial characteristics have been shown to have significant associations with OSA/SDB [41]. A narrow or retrusive maxilla, retrognathic mandible, hyperdivergent mandibular plane angle, steep palatal plane angle, increased lower face height, decreased ratio of posterior to anterior face heights, anterior open bite, obtuse gonial angle, obtuse cranial base angle, and inferior position of the hyoid bone have been shown to be associated with pediatric OSA [41–47]. Arthritic involvement of the TMJ and the resulting retrognathia/micrognathia might be related to the increased OSA prevalence in JIA patients, as both are common in JIA, and both are risk factors for OSA [48,49].

Attended PSG is one of the more predictable methods to diagnose OSA [39]. The prevalence of OSA determined by varying AHI thresholds in PSG in the general pediatric population is 1–4% [50]. Limited data exists to determine the prevalence of SDB/OSA problems in JIA patients, but it has been demonstrated that 40% of children with JIA had an AHI of greater than or equal to 1.5 events per hour, as measured by PSG [36,51]. Pain, fatigue, and medication side effects are often attributed to causing sleep disturbances in JIA patients without screening for underlying OSA, and the average time from the diagnosis of JIA to the discovery of OSA (when present) by PSG is 2.5 years, which may be significant given the complications of OSA in overall health and disease management [49]. Most JIA patients with OSA are undiagnosed and untreated, which likely contributes to a poorer treatment response and worse patient-reported outcomes [36].

As the potential craniofacial morphology alterations associated with TMJ arthritis in JIA patients closely resemble those commonly associated with airway compromise in pediatric patients, it is of particular interest to investigate potential airway-related sequalae of JIA. At present, there are no known published studies that evaluate upper airway dimensions in JIA patients using three-dimensional CBCT data. The purpose of this study is to evaluate upper airway volumes, the most constricted cross-sectional areas, and cephalometric values in JIA patients and compare them to healthy controls to determine if any differences exist.

2. Subject and Methods

This study is a retrospective case control study evaluating patients with and without JIA. Ethical approval was obtained from the University of Alabama Institutional Review Board #30000975. Patients presenting in the Orthodontic department at the University of Alabama School of Dentistry from 2018–2021 were reviewed. JIA patient had the following records: (1) MRI of the TMJ, (2) clinical photographs, and (3) a CBCT with a field of view that included the TMJ. A brief status of the JIA patients was also recorded. Patients who presented for orthodontic treatment and had clinical photographs and a CBCT were eligible as control patients. The control group was carefully selected to be age matched to the JIA group. Control patients were excluded from the study if they had any of the following characteristics: (1) history of arthritis, immune disease, or systemic disease confirmed by or under investigation by a rheumatologist, (2) history of diagnosed TMJ dysfunction, (3) congenital syndromes, or (4) craniofacial trauma.

The JIA study group comprised of 32 patients with a mean age of 13.6 years, consisting of 10 males and 22 females. The control group comprised 32 patients with a mean age of 13.75 years, consisting of 13 males and 19 females.

2.1. CBCT Acquisition

The CBCT image volumes for all JIA and control patients were captured using the same Carestream 9300 CBCT machine (Carestream Dental, Atlanta, GA, USA). The CBCT scan time was 14 s with a radiation dose of 20 μSi and image resolution up to 0.90 μm. Each image was saved in the universal Digital Imaging and Communications in Medicine or DICOM (*.dcm) format. Each image was imported into Dolphin Imaging software (Version 11.95 Premium, Dolphin Imaging & Management Solutions, Chatsworth, GA, USA). All images were oriented to the Frankfurt horizontal (FH) plane in the sagittal dimension and by leveling the right and left orbitale points in the frontal dimension.

2.2. Cephalometric Rendering and Analysis

Dolphin Imaging software was used to render a cephalometric image for each patient from the CBCT DICOM data. Each cephalometric image was generated from the algorithm proprietary to the imaging software and produced an orthogonal perspective with 0% magnification. The cephalometric image was digitally traced, and the following values were identified: sella-nasion-A point (SNA) angle, sella-nasion-B point (SNB) angle, A point-nasion-B point (ANB) angle, anterior facial height (AFH), posterior facial height (PFH), PFH to AFH ratio, mandibular plane angle (SN-MP), FMA (FH-MP), overjet (OJ), and overbite (OB). See Figure 1.

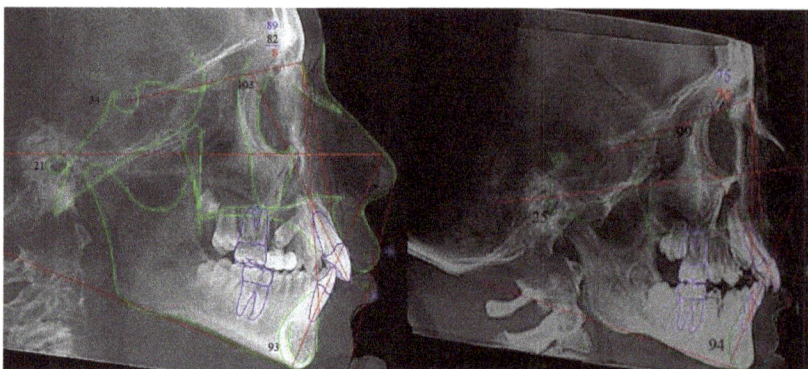

Figure 1. Cephalometric images rendered from CBCT DICOM data and traced using Dolphin Imaging. The (**left**) is a patient from the control group and the (**right**) is a patient from the JIA group.

2.3. Airway Measurements

The sinus/airway module of Dolphin Imaging was used to segment the three-dimensional representation of the upper airway, as well as determine the most constricted cross-sectional area (MCCA) of the upper airway. The inferior boundary of the oropharynx was set as a horizonal line from the anterior–superior corner of the third cervical vertebrae (C3), and the superior boundary was determined as a horizontal line from the posterior nasal spine (PNS). The nasopharynx extended from the superior limit of the oropharynx (PNS-horizontal) to a line extending vertically from PNS (PNS-vertical). The airway sensitivity in the Dolphin Imaging software was determined based on the most accurate visual rendering of the proper airway volume in our study groups and was set to 30 (on a scale from 0 to 100) for all patients. The MCCA was found within either the oropharynx or nasopharynx using the "minimal axial area" feature built into the Dolphin Imaging software. All measurements were done by a single investigator. A second investigator (MG) analyzed the airways of a random sample of 10 study patients. See Figure 2.

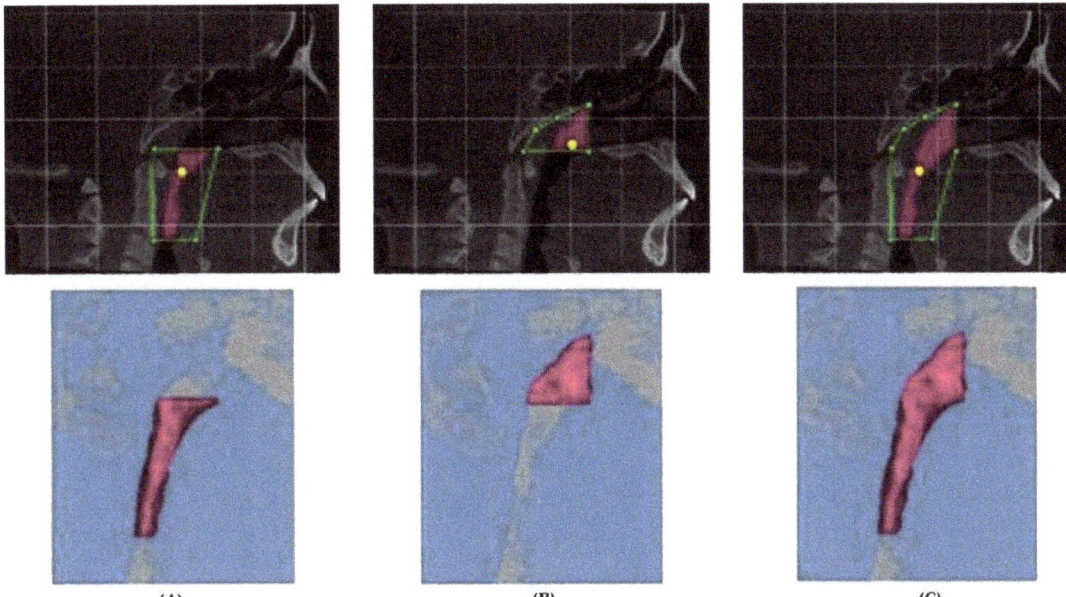

Figure 2. Showing boundaries of airway segmentation performed in Dolphin Imaging for (**A**) oropharynx, (**B**) nasopharynx, and (**C**) total upper airway.

2.4. Statistical Analysis

All data were entered onto an Excel spreadsheet. The datasets for each individual reading were tested and analyzed and found to be normally distributed. A Student's unpaired *t*-test was performed to compare airway volumes, MCCA values, and cephalometric values between the JIA patients and control group. In addition, the ODDs ratio was calculated. This analysis was used to determine the measure of association between a particular variable and the group measured.

3. Results

The results of each variable measured are presented on Table 1. Data from the first and second investigators were analyzed using a *t*-test, and no statistical differences were found. In addition, the data collected from each investigator had a high degree of reproducibility, indicating that the airway variables measured were reliable and accurate for analysis.

Table 1. Mean and standard deviation of each variable in control and JIA study groups, as well as *p*-value for statistical significance of unpaired Student *t*-test. In addition, the ODDS ratio was also calculated. * Indicates statistical significance.

Variable	Control Mean (SD)	JIA Mean (SD)	*p*-Value Mean (SD)	ODDS Ratio (Confidence Range)
Age (years)	13.75 (2.91)	13.59 (2.73)	0.825	1
SNA (Degrees)	83.06 (3.45)	81.53 (4.27)	0.12	1.00 (0.42–2.35)
SNB (Degrees)	79.29 (3.65)	78.43 (4.42)	0.398	0.88 (0.32–2.44)
ANB (Degrees)	3.69 (2.84)	3.21 (2.15)	0.448	0.45 (0.16–1.25)
Anterior Face Height(mm)	113.12 (9.46)	109.16 (8.51)	0.083	0.72 (0.23–2.23)
Posterior Face Height (mm)	75.39 (7.05)	71.06 (7.87)	0.024 *	5.40 (1.66–17.56) *
PFH/AFH Ratio	66.58 (5.67)	65.12 (5.08)	0.281	1.29 (0.48–3.44)
SN-MP (Degrees)	32.45 (7.30)	33.51 (6.12)	0.529	0.85 (0.28–2.59)

Table 1. Cont.

Variable	Control Mean (SD)	JIA Mean (SD)	p-Value Mean (SD)	ODDS Ratio (Confidence Range)
FMA (Degrees)	22.97 (7.33)	22.88 (5.79)	0.958	1 (0.34–2.97)
Overbite (mm)	2.81 (2.37)	2.13 (1.28)	0.159	0.77 (0.15–3.53)
Overjet (mm)	4.15 (2.33)	4.43 (3.90)	0.734	0.68 (0.25–1.84)
Oropharynx Airway Volume (mm^3)	14,047.31 (5586.36)	11,098.03 (6268.15)	0.051	3.40 (1.18–9.81) *
Nasopharynx Airway Volume (mm^3)	5827.03 (2425.85)	4392.19 (1203.04)	0.004 *	4.59 (1.54–13.67) *
Total Upper Airway Volume (mm^3)	19,874.34 (6790.35)	15,490.22 (6945.79)	0.013 *	3.22 (0.77–13.50) *
Minimal Cross-Sectional Area (mm^2)	202.50 (103.03)	143.75 (103.23)	0.026 *	2.96 (0.95–9.21) *

3.1. Cephalometric Analysis

The cephalometric variables were compared between the JIA study group and the control group. Only the variable of the posterior facial height was found to be statistically and significantly different between the two groups, measuring 71.06 mm in the JIA group and 75.39 mm in the control group ($p < 0.05$). The ODDs ratio confirmed the posterior facial height to be significantly smaller in the JIA group.

3.2. Airway Analysis

The airway variables were compared between the JIA study group and the control group. The JIA sample was significantly different than the control group for the following airway parameters. The total upper airway volume (nasopharynx and oropharynx combined) was 15,490 mm^3 in the JIA group and 19,874 mm^3 in the control group ($p < 0.05$). The nasopharynx volume was 4392 mm^3 in the JIA group and 5827 mm^3 in the control group ($p < 0.01$). The oropharynx volume in the JIA group was 11,098 mm^3 compared to 14,047 mm^3 in the control group, which was close to but did not quite reach statistical significance ($p = 0.051$). The MCCA was 144 mm^2 in the JIA group and 203 mm^2 in the control group ($p < 0.05$). The ODDs ratio also indicated a significant association of JIA patients with the variables measured in all the airway analysis.

4. Discussion

The JIA and control groups being evaluated were age-matched ($p = 0.825$) to account for normal growth-related changes in cephalometric and airway parameters [52]. The cephalometric values evaluated allowed for the study of the anteroposterior and vertical craniofacial morphologies, which are of interest in this study because there is evidence that anteroposterior jaw positions and mandibular posterior rotation can affect the airway.

4.1. Cephalometric Parameters

Many previous studies have documented differences in cephalometric variables between JIA patients and control patients [5,6,13,15,21–27]. However, our data did not demonstrate statistically significant differences in cephalometric values between the two groups in any variable other than posterior facial height ($p = 0.024$). A difference in the posterior facial height has been previously demonstrated in other studies [13,15,23]. One possible explanation for the lack of differences in cephalometric values could be that the control group represented an already retrognathic sample. It does appear that both our JIA and control groups have a tendency toward mild mandibular retrognathia, with the ANB angles of the JIA group and control group measured at 3.21 and 3.69 degrees, respectively. Additionally, the absence of cephalometric differences between the groups may suggest that the treatment regimens employed in the treatment of JIA patients were effective at minimizing craniofacial growth disturbances secondary to JIA.

4.2. Airway Parameters

Previous studies have demonstrated that groups with different craniofacial growth patterns have shown differences in CBCT-derived airway parameters [53–57]. Interestingly, despite minimal cephalometric differences between our two groups, we did find statistically significant differences in nasopharyngeal airway volume (NAV), total upper airway volume (TUAV), and MCCA. In the JIA group, 16 of 32 patients (50%) had an MCA of less than 100 mm^2, while the control group had only 6 of 32 patients (18.75%) with an MCA less than 100 mm^2. The value of 100 mm^2 was chosen because it roughly represents the lowest quarter (25%) of the range of MCCA values that were found in both our JIA and control groups, as well as being easy to visually identify using Dolphin Imaging. In addition, the oropharyngeal airway volume (OAV) difference between the groups approached statistical significance (p = 0.051). Another possible question that arose from this study was "Could the posterior face height be a significant factor in airway volume and MCCA?". However, this seems unlikely given the difference in posterior face height between the two groups was 4.33 mm, which represents about 5% of the average posterior face height of 71.06 mm in the JIA group. However, the 2D representation of the cephalogram does not take into account the 3D anatomical dentofacial deformity present in some JIA patients (Figure 3). Finally, evidence of sleep-disordered breathing (SDB) has been previously shown in JIA patients that have no evidence of cervical spine or TMJ arthritis [48]. At present, not enough information is available to investigate other reasons as to why airway parameters were different between the two groups. However, based on our data, it does appear that additional factors other than craniofacial morphology may contribute to the anatomic airway reduction in JIA patients. In the general pediatric population, other factors that could contribute to airway compromise include obesity, size of adenoids and tonsils, and presence of allergic rhinitis [42,58–66].

Anatomic and structural features alone are certainly part of the overall pathogenesis of SDB and OSA [60]. However, the fact that patients with OSA do not have airway compromise when awake demonstrates that there is more to the picture than just anatomy, and in fact, upper airway neuromuscular tone plays a large role in normal respiratory patency and function [67]. Additionally, children have been shown to have a reduced tendency toward cortical arousals that would otherwise correct for obstructions that occur during sleep [67]. Nevertheless, correlations between CBCT-derived airway dimensions and AHI have been shown, demonstrating that airway anatomy is a definite factor in airway compromise during sleep and that CBCT should be viewed as a useful tool in evaluating the airway in pediatric patients [34,35]. That being said, CBCT airway analysis certainly has its limitations. A CBCT image provides a representation of the airway at only one static time point of the respiratory cycle with the patient in an upright and awake posture. Additionally, there is evidence that successive CBCT images taken on the same patient only a few months apart are prone to considerable variations in airway volumes [68].

Visual inspection of the 3D airway morphology revealed an interesting finding that requires further investigation from a larger sample. Of the 32 patients with JIA, 21 demonstrated asymmetric deviations of the airway form when evaluated from the 3D frontal view of the airway volume. This represented 67% of the patients reviewed. It is not uncommon for a JIA patient population to also show facial asymmetries when evaluating skeletal and soft tissue forms, but to be able to visualize this in a 3D manner was revolutionary (Figure 4). Further work is required in evaluating for the presence of a correlation between the skeletal/facial and airway asymmetries.

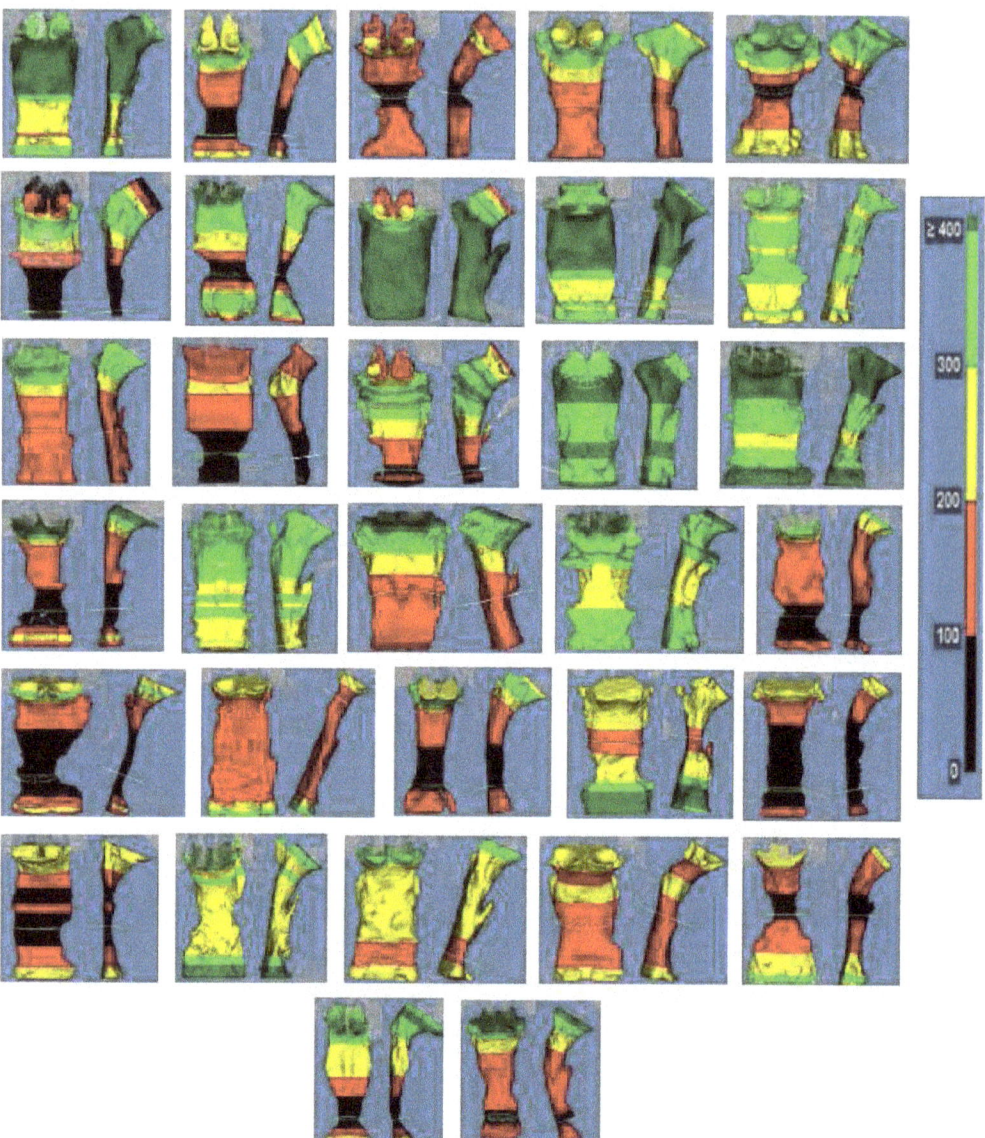

Figure 3. Frontal and sagittal views of the airways of all JIA patients with the scale measured in square millimeters of airway cross-section and a marker showing the level of the minimal cross-sectional area of each. Please note that visualizing the color map of the airway utilizes a different feature of Dolphin Imaging, which does not allow for as much precision in setting the upper and lower airway boundaries and is only used here to give a visual representation of the cross-sectional areas at different levels of the airway. All quantitative volumetric and minimal cross-sectional data were gathered with the segmentation boundaries set, as described in Section 2 and as shown in Figure 2.

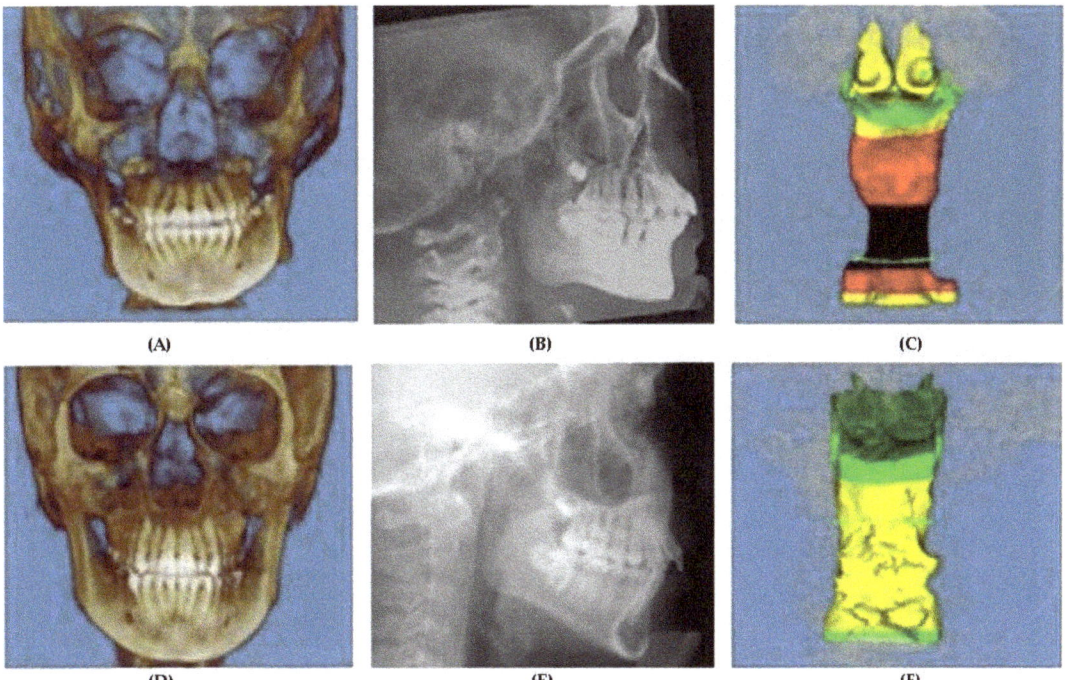

Figure 4. (**A–C**) Images from a JIA patient with a chin deviation to the left side and an asymmetric airway with a "twist" effect. (**D–F**) Images of a control patient representative of the control group with no skeletal asymmetry and an airway with no gross asymmetries.

4.3. Software Analysis and Interpretations

When evaluating the software programs commercially available for airway analysis of the CBCT DICOM data, some positive and negative qualities have been noted. Dolphin Imaging, which was used in our study, has been validated as having high reliability in measuring the airway consistently between repeated measurements of the same image data and when comparing two airways when both were measured with Dolphin Imaging [69]. For this reason, the data obtained for the JIA and control groups in our study have a high level of validity, given that the airways were all rendered with Dolphin Imaging using the same technique and by the same operator. However, these same software programs, including Dolphin Imaging, have been shown to have poor accuracy when comparing the airway volume values between different software programs [69]. This finding, combined with the fact that there are not currently clear segmentation standards for landmarks used to define the upper and lower boundaries of the different subdivisions of the upper airway, make it difficult to compare airway volumes from one study to another or to use proposed normative values to evaluate study results or individual patients.

4.4. JIA, Airway and OSA

Timely diagnosis of TMJ arthritis in JIA patients is critical to allow for early intervention and to reduce the risk of any possible craniofacial growth alterations. Our study demonstrated a reduced airway dimension in JIA patients, and this finding may have an effect on OSA. Due to the significant influences that OSA may have in overall health and disease management, early identification of debilitating craniofacial effects of JIA is critical. Referral for orthodontic evaluation of the craniofacial structures may provide additional information useful in evaluating OSA risk factors. While CBCT images cannot provide a diagnosis of OSA, they may be a useful screening tool. Additionally, there is evidence that screening JIA patients with the Pediatric Sleep Questionnaire (PSQ) could lead to a timelier diagnosis and treatment of SDB [36].

4.5. Study Limitations

Our study is unique in that no one has previously demonstrated 3D airway differences in a JIA patient population. However, our study did have a number of limitations. The retrospective study design does not allow for ideal standardization of the CBCT acquisitions. Not all CBCT images were taken by a single operator, which may have some effect on optimal patient positioning. Additionally, there was no ability to make sure that all patients were given the same instructions for breathing and tongue posture instructions during the image acquisition. Additionally, when considering selection of patients for the control group, it is not standard protocol in our clinic to have a CBCT image taken for all patients undergoing orthodontic evaluation, and CBCT images are often acquired when there is an out-of-the-ordinary finding, dentofacial diagnostic need, or suspicion. For this reason, it is possible that our control group consisted of patients that are not a true representation of the standard norm. During the segmentation of the airway, a common threshold value was used for all patients, while other authors have discussed using an "interactive" method of setting the threshold value in which the threshold is determined for each patient individually at a number that provides a visual best fit of the airway. However, there is no evidence to suspect that our segmentation method created errors on any individual scans.

5. Conclusions

The following conclusions were obtained from this study:

(1). There was a difference in the posterior face height between JIA and control patients.
(2). There was a significant difference in total upper airway volume, nasopharynx airway volume, and most constricted cross-sectional area measurements between JIA and control patients.
(3). The ODDs ratio analysis confirmed the association of the statistically significant parameters above.
(4). 50% of JIA patients had an airway with a most constricted cross-sectional area of less than 100 mm^2.
(5). 67% of JIA patients had an asymmetric airway form.

Author Contributions: Conceptualization, C.H.K.; formal analysis, M.G., M.L.S., T.P. and C.H.K.; investigation, R.Q.C. and B.E.K.; methodology, M.G. and C.H.K.; project administration, T.P. and C.H.K.; writing—original draft, M.G. and C.H.K.; writing—review and editing, R.Q.C. and M.L.S. All authors have read and agreed to the published version of the manuscript.

Funding: Biomedical Research Award, American Association of Orthodontics Foundation.

Institutional Review Board Statement: University of Alabama at Birmingham Institutional Review Board gave approval for the study. IRB#30000975.

Informed Consent Statement: Informed consent was obtained from all patients in the study.

Data Availability Statement: Data is available at the UAB Department of Orthodontics repository.

Conflicts of Interest: The authors declare no conflict of interest.

References

1. Crayne, C.B.; Beukelman, T. Juvenile Idiopathic Arthritis: Oligoarthritis and Polyarthritis. *Pediatr Clin. N. Am.* **2018**, *65*, 657–674. [CrossRef]
2. Prakken, B.; Albani, S.; Martini, A. Juvenile idiopathic arthritis. *Lancet* **2011**, *377*, 2138–2149. [CrossRef]
3. Bukovac, L.T.; Perica, M. Juvenile Idiopathic Arthritis. *Reumatizam* **2016**, *63* (Suppl. 1), 53–58.
4. Hersh, A.O.; Prahalad, S. Immunogenetics of juvenile idiopathic arthritis: A comprehensive review. *J. Autoimmun.* **2015**, *64*, 113–124. [CrossRef]

5. Ringold, S.; Cron, R.Q. The temporomandibular joint in juvenile idiopathic arthritis: Frequently used and frequently arthritic. *Pediatr. Rheumatol.* **2009**, *7*, 11. [CrossRef]
6. Twilt, M.; Schulten, A.J.M.; Nicolaas, P.; Dülger, A.; van Suijlekom-Smit, L.W. Facioskeletal changes in children with juvenile idiopathic arthritis. *Ann. Rheum. Dis.* **2006**, *65*, 823–825. [CrossRef]
7. Kau, C.H.; Allareddy, V.; Stoustrup, P.; Pedersen, T.; Kinard, B.; Cron, R.Q.; Stoll, M.L.; Gilbert, G.H. Management of juvenile idiopathic arthritis: Preliminary qualitative findings from the National Dental Practice-Based Research Network. *J. World Fed. Orthod.* **2021**, *10*, 70–73. [CrossRef]
8. Abramowicz, S.; Levy, J.M.; Prahalad, S.; Travers, C.D.; Angeles-Han, S. Temporomandibular joint involvement in children with juvenile idiopathic arthritis: A preliminary report. *Oral Surg. Oral Med. Oral Pathol. Oral Radiol.* **2019**, *127*, 19–23. [CrossRef]
9. Arabshahi, B.; Cron, R. Temporomandibular joint arthritis in juvenile idiopathic arthritis: The forgotten joint. *Curr. Opin. Rheumatol.* **2006**, *18*, 490–495. [CrossRef]
10. Pawlaczyk-Kamieńska, T.; Paczyk-Wróblewskawla, E.; Borysewicz-Lewicka, M. Early diagnosis of temporomandibular joint arthritis in children with juvenile idiopathic arthritis. A systematic review. *Eur. J. Paediatr. Dent.* **2020**, *21*, 219–226.
11. Stoll, M.L.; Kau, C.H.; Waite, P.D.; Cron, R.Q. Temporomandibular joint arthritis in juvenile idiopathic arthritis, now what? *Pediatr. Rheumatol.* **2018**, *16*, 32. [CrossRef]
12. Abramowicz, S.; Kim, S.; Prahalad, S.; Chouinard, A.-F.; Kaban, L.B. Juvenile arthritis: Current concepts in terminology, etiopathogenesis, diagnosis, and management. *Int. J. Oral Maxillofac. Surg.* **2016**, *45*, 801–812. [CrossRef]
13. Billiau, A.D.; Hu, Y.; Verdonck, A.; Carels, C.; Wouters, C. Temporomandibular joint arthritis in juvenile idiopathic arthritis: Prevalence, clinical and radiological signs, and relation to dentofacial morphology. *J. Rheumatol.* **2007**, *34*, 1925–1933.
14. Abramowicz, S.; Susarla, H.K.; Kim, S.; Kaban, L.B. Physical Findings Associated with Active Temporomandibular Joint Inflammation in Children with Juvenile Idiopathic Arthritis. *J. Oral Maxillofac. Surg.* **2013**, *71*, 1683–1687. [CrossRef]
15. Stabrun, A.E.; Larheim, T.A.; Höyeraal, H.M.; Rösler, M. Reduced mandibular dimensions and asymmetry in juvenile rheumatoid arthritis. Pathogenetic factors. *Arthritis Rheum.* **1988**, *31*, 602–611. [CrossRef]
16. Koos, B.; Twilt, M.; Kyank, U.; Fischer-Brandies, H.; Gaßling, V.; Tzaribachev, N. Reliability of Clinical Symptoms in Diagnosing Temporomandibular Joint Arthritis in Juvenile Idiopathic Arthritis. *J. Rheumatol.* **2014**, *41*, 1871–1877. [CrossRef]
17. Pedersen, T.K.; Küseler, A.; Gelineck, J.; Herlin, T. A prospective study of magnetic resonance and radiographic imaging in relation to symptoms and clinical findings of the temporomandibular joint in children with juvenile idiopathic arthritis. *J. Rheumatol.* **2008**, *35*, 1668–1675.
18. Celebi, A.A.; Cron, R.; Stoll, M.; Simsek, S.; Kinard, B.; Waite, P.D.; Wang, J.; Vo, V.; Tran, L.; Kau, C.H. Comparison of the condyle-fossa relationship and resorption between patients with and without Juvenile Idiopathic Ar-thritis (JIA). *J. Oral Maxillofac. Surg.* **2022**, *80*, 422–430. [CrossRef]
19. Twilt, M.; Mobers, S.M.L.M.; Arends, L.R.; Cate, R.T.; Van Suijlekom-Smit, L. Temporomandibular involvement in juvenile idiopathic arthritis. *J. Rheumatol.* **2004**, *31*, 1418–1422. [CrossRef]
20. Kristensen, K.D.; Stoustrup, P.; Küseler, A.; Pedersen, T.K.; Twilt, M.; Herlin, T. Clinical predictors of temporomandibular joint arthritis in juvenile idiopathic arthritis: A systematic literature review. *Semin. Arthritis Rheum.* **2016**, *45*, 717–732. [CrossRef]
21. Weiss, P.F.; Arabshahi, B.; Johnson, A.; Bilaniuk, L.T.; Zarnow, D.; Cahill, A.M.; Feudtner, C.; Cron, R. High prevalence of temporomandibular joint arthritis at disease onset in children with juvenile idiopathic arthritis, as detected by magnetic resonance imaging but not by ultrasound. *Arthritis Rheum.* **2008**, *58*, 1189–1196. [CrossRef]
22. Koos, B.; Gassling, V.; Bott, S.; Tzaribachev, N.; Godt, A. Pathological changes in the TMJ and the length of the ramus in patients with confirmed juvenile idiopathic arthritis. *J. Cranio -Maxillofac. Surg.* **2014**, *42*, 1802–1807. [CrossRef]
23. Piancino, M.G.; Cannavale, R.; Dalmasso, P.; Tonni, I.; Garagiola, U.; Perillo, L.; Olivieri, A.N. Cranial structure and condylar asymmetry of patients with juvenile idiopathic arthritis: A risky growth pattern. *Clin. Rheumatol.* **2018**, *37*, 2667–2673. [CrossRef]
24. Hsieh, Y.-J.; Darvann, T.A.; Hermann, N.V.; Larsen, P.; Liao, Y.-F.; Bjoern-Joergensen, J.; Kreiborg, S. Facial morphology in children and adolescents with juvenile idiopathic arthritis and moderate to severe temporomandibular joint involvement. *Am. J. Orthod. Dentofac. Orthop.* **2016**, *149*, 182–191. [CrossRef]
25. Kjellberg, H.; Fasth, A.; Kiliaridis, S.; Wenneberg, B.; Thilander, B. Craniofacial structure in children with juvenile chronic arthritis (JCA) compared with healthy children with ideal or postnormal occlusion. *Am. J. Orthod. Dentofac. Orthop.* **1995**, *107*, 67–78. [CrossRef]
26. Kjellberg, H. Juvenile chronic arthritis. Dentofacial morphology, growth, mandibular function and orthodontic treatment. *Swed. Dent. J. Suppl.* **1995**, *109*, 1–56.
27. Sidiropoulou-Chatzigianni, S.; Papadopoulos, M.A.; Kolokithas, G. Dentoskeletal Morphology in Children with Juvenile Idiopathic Arthritis Compared with Healthy Children. *J. Orthod.* **2001**, *28*, 53–58. [CrossRef]
28. Srivastava, K.C.; Shrivastava, D.; Austin, R.D. Journey towards the 3D dental imaging—The milestones in the advancement of dental imaging. *Int. J. Adv. Res.* **2016**, *4*, 377–382. [CrossRef]
29. Ogawa, T.; Enciso, R.; Shintaku, W.H.; Clark, G.T. Evaluation of cross-section airway configuration of obstructive sleep apnea. *Oral Surg. Oral Med. Oral Pathol. Oral Radiol. Endodontol.* **2007**, *103*, 102–108. [CrossRef]
30. Enciso, R.; Nguyen, M.; Shigeta, Y.; Ogawa, T.; Clark, G.T. Comparison of cone-beam CT parameters and sleep questionnaires in sleep apnea patients and control subjects. *Oral Surg. Oral Med. Oral Pathol. Oral Radiol. Endodontol.* **2010**, *109*, 285–293. [CrossRef]

31. Buchanan, A.; Cohen, R.; Looney, S.; Kalathingal, S.; De Rossi, S. Cone-beam CT analysis of patients with obstructive sleep apnea compared to normal controls. *Imaging Sci. Dent.* **2016**, *46*, 9–16. [CrossRef]
32. Momany, S.M.; AlJamal, G.; Shugaa-Addin, B.; Khader, Y.S. Cone Beam Computed Tomography Analysis of Upper Airway Measurements in Patients with Obstructive Sleep Apnea. *Am. J. Med. Sci.* **2016**, *352*, 376–384. [CrossRef]
33. Tikku, T.; Khanna, R.; Sachan, K.; Agarwal, A.; Srivastava, K.; Lal, A. Dimensional and volumetric analysis of the oropharyngeal region in obstructive sleep apnea patients: A cone beam computed tomography study. *Dent. Res. J.* **2016**, *13*, 396–404.
34. Hsu, W.; Kang, K.; Yao, C.J.; Chou, C.; Weng, W.; Lee, P.; Chen, Y. Evaluation of Upper Airway in Children with Obstructive Sleep Apnea Using Cone-Beam Computed Tomography. *Laryngoscope* **2021**, *131*, 680–685. [CrossRef]
35. Masoud, A.I.; Alwadei, A.H.; Gowharji, L.F.; Park, C.G.; Carley, D.W. Relating three-dimensional airway measurements to the apnea-hypopnea index in pediatric sleep apnea patients. *Orthod. Craniofac. Res.* **2021**, *24*, 137–146. [CrossRef]
36. Ward, T.M.; Chen, M.L.; Landis, C.A.; Ringold, S.; Beebe, D.W.; Pike, K.C.; Wallace, C.A. Congruence between polysomnography obstructive sleep apnea and the pediatric sleep questionnaire: Fatigue and health-related quality of life in juvenile idiopathic arthritis. *Qual. Life Res.* **2017**, *26*, 779–788. [CrossRef]
37. Tarakçı, E.; Arman, N.; Barut, K.; Şahin, S.; Adroviç, A.; Kasapçopur, Ö. Fatigue and sleep in children and adolescents with juvenile idiopathic arthritis: A cross-sectional study. *Turk. J. Med. Sci.* **2019**, *49*, 58–65. [CrossRef]
38. Armbrust, W.; Siers, N.E.; Lelieveld, O.T.; Mouton, L.J.; Tuinstra, J.; Sauer, P. Fatigue in patients with juvenile idiopathic arthritis: A systematic review of the literature. *Semin. Arthritis Rheum.* **2016**, *45*, 587–595. [CrossRef]
39. Trosman, I.; Trosman, S.J. Cognitive and Behavioral Consequences of Sleep Disordered Breathing in Children. *Med. Sci.* **2017**, *5*, 30. [CrossRef]
40. Guilleminault, C.; Korobkin, R.; Winkle, R. A review of 50 children with obstructive sleep apnea syndrome. *Lung* **1981**, *159*, 275–287. [CrossRef]
41. Özdemir, H.; Altin, R.; Söğüt, A.; Çınar, F.; Mahmutyazıcıoğlu, K.; Kart, L.; Uzun, L.; Davşancı, H.; Gündoğdu, S.; Tomaç, N. Craniofacial differences according to AHI scores of children with obstructive sleep apnoea syndrome: Cephalometric study in 39 patients. *Pediatr. Radiol.* **2004**, *34*, 393–399.
42. Katz, E.S.; D'Ambrosio, C.M. Pathophysiology of Pediatric Obstructive Sleep Apnea. *Proc. Am. Thorac. Soc.* **2008**, *5*, 253–262. [CrossRef]
43. Galeotti, A.; Festa, P.; Viarani, V.; Pavone, M.; Sitzia, E.; Piga, S.; Cutrera, R.; De Vincentiis, G.; D'Antò, V. Correlation between cephalometric variables and obstructive sleep apnoea severity in children. *Eur. J. Paediatr. Dent.* **2019**, *20*, 43–47. [PubMed]
44. Joseph, A.; Elbaum, J.; Cisneros, G.J.; Eisig, S.B. A cephalometric comparative study of the soft tissue airway dimensions in persons with hyperdivergent and normodivergent facial patterns. *J. Oral Maxillofac. Surg.* **1998**, *56*, 135–139; discussion 139–140. [CrossRef]
45. Flores-Mir, C.; Korayem, M.; Heo, G.; Witmans, M.; Major, M.P.; Major, P.W. Craniofacial morphological characteristics in children with obstructive sleep apnea syndrome: A systematic review and meta-analysis. *J. Am. Dent. Assoc.* **2013**, *144*, 269–277. [CrossRef] [PubMed]
46. Katyal, V.; Pamula, Y.; Martin, A.J.; Daynes, C.N.; Kennedy, J.D.; Sampson, W.J. Craniofacial and upper airway morphology in pediatric sleep-disordered breathing: Systematic review and meta-analysis. *Am. J. Orthod. Dentofac. Orthop.* **2013**, *143*, 20–30.e3. [CrossRef]
47. Kawashima, S.; Niikuni, N.; Chia-Hung, L.; Takahasi, Y.; Kohno, M.; Nakajima, I.; Akasaka, M.; Sakata, H.; Akashi, S. Cephalometric Comparisons of Craniofacial and Upper Airway Structures in Young Children with Obstructive Sleep Apnea Syndrome. *Ear Nose Throat J.* **2000**, *79*, 499–502, 505–506. [CrossRef]
48. Bloom, B.J.; Owens, J.A.; McGuinn, M.; Nobile, C.; Schaeffer, L.; Alario, A.J. Sleep and its relationship to pain, dysfunction, and disease activity in juvenile rheumatoid arthritis. *J. Rheumatol.* **2002**, *29*, 169–173.
49. Ward, T.M.; Beebe, D.W.; Chen, M.L.; Landis, C.A.; Ringold, S.; Pike, K.; Wallace, C.A. Sleep Disturbances and Neurobehavioral Performance in Juvenile Idiopathic Arthritis. *J. Rheumatol.* **2017**, *44*, 361–367. [CrossRef]
50. Lumeng, J.C.; Chervin, R.D. Epidemiology of Pediatric Obstructive Sleep Apnea. *Proc. Am. Thorac. Soc.* **2008**, *5*, 242–252. [CrossRef]
51. Ward, T.M.; Archbold, K.; Lentz, M.; Ringold, S.; Wallace, C.A.; Landis, C.A. Sleep Disturbance, Daytime Sleepiness, and Neurocognitive Performance in Children with Juvenile Idiopathic Arthritis. *Sleep* **2010**, *33*, 252–259. [CrossRef]
52. Schendel, S.A.; Jacobson, R.; Khalessi, S. Airway Growth and Development: A Computerized 3-Dimensional Analysis. *J. Oral Maxillofac. Surg.* **2012**, *70*, 2174–2183. [CrossRef] [PubMed]
53. Nath, M.; Ahmed, J.; Ongole, R.; Denny, C.; Shenoy, N. CBCT analysis of pharyngeal airway volume and comparison of airway volume among patients with skeletal Class I, Class II, and Class III malocclusion: A retrospective study. *Cranio* **2021**, *39*, 379–390. [CrossRef] [PubMed]
54. Alhammadi, M.S.; Almashraqi, A.A.; Halboub, E.; Almahdi, S.; Jali, T.; Atafi, A.; Alomar, F. Pharyngeal airway spaces in different skeletal malocclusions: A CBCT 3D assessment. *Cranio* **2021**, *39*, 97–106. [CrossRef] [PubMed]
55. Wang, X.; Chen, H.; Jia, L.; Xu, X.; Guo, J. The relationship between three-dimensional craniofacial and upper airway anatomical variables and severity of obstructive sleep apnoea in adults. *Eur. J. Orthod.* **2021**, *44*, 78–85. [CrossRef]
56. Tseng, Y.-C.; Tsai, F.-C.; Chou, S.-T.; Hsu, C.-Y.; Cheng, J.-H.; Chen, C.-M. Evaluation of pharyngeal airway volume for different dentofacial skeletal patterns using cone-beam computed tomography. *J. Dent. Sci.* **2021**, *16*, 51–57. [CrossRef]

57. Castro-Silva, L.; Monnazzi, M.S.; Spin-Neto, R.; de Moraes, M.; Miranda, S.; Gabrielli, M.F.R.; Filho, V.P. Cone-beam evaluation of pharyngeal airway space in class I, II, and III patients. *Oral Surg. Oral Med. Oral Pathol. Oral Radiol.* **2015**, *120*, 679–683. [CrossRef]
58. Redline, S.; Tishler, P.V.; Schluchter, M.; Aylor, J.; Clark, K.; Graham, G. Risk Factors for Sleep-disordered Breathing in Children. Associations with obesity, race, and respiratory problems.Children. *Am. J. Respir. Crit. Care Med.* **1999**, *159 Pt 1*, 1527–1532. [CrossRef]
59. Marcus, C.L.; Brooks, L.J.; Draper, K.A.; Gozal, D.; Halbower, A.C.; Jones, J.; Schechter, M.S.; Ward, S.D.; Sheldon, S.H.; Shiffman, R.N. Diagnosis and management of childhood obstructive sleep apnea syndrome. *Pediatrics* **2012**, *130*, 576–584. [CrossRef]
60. Isono, S.; Shimada, A.; Utsugi, M.; Konno, A.; Nishino, T. Comparison of static mechanical properties of the passive pharynx be-tween normal children and children with sleep-disordered breathing. *Am. J. Respir. Crit. Care Med.* **1998**, *157 Pt 1*, 1204–1212. [CrossRef]
61. Lin, S.Y.; Melvin, T.-A.N.; Boss, E.F.; Ishman, S.L. The association between allergic rhinitis and sleep-disordered breathing in children: A systematic review. *Int. Forum Allergy Rhinol.* **2013**, *3*, 504–509. [CrossRef]
62. Cao, Y.; Wu, S.; Zhang, L.; Yang, Y.; Cao, S.; Li, Q. Association of allergic rhinitis with obstructive sleep apnea: A meta-analysis. *Medicine* **2018**, *97*, e13783. [CrossRef] [PubMed]
63. Gileles-Hillel, A.; Alonso-Álvarez, M.L.; Gozal, L.; Peris, E.; Cordero-Guevara, J.A.; Terán-Santos, J.; Martinez, M.G.; Jurado-Luque, M.J.; Corral-Peñafiel, J.; Duran-Cantolla, J.; et al. Inflammatory markers and obstructive sleep apnea in obese children: The NANOS study. *Mediat. Inflamm.* **2014**, *2014*, 605280. [CrossRef] [PubMed]
64. Tam, C.S.; Wong, M.; McBain, R.; Bailey, S.; Waters, K.A. Inflammatory measures in children with obstructive sleep apnoea. *J. Paediatr. Child. Health* **2006**, *42*, 277–282. [CrossRef] [PubMed]
65. Küseler, A.; Pedersen, T.K.; Gelineck, J.; Herlin, T. A 2 year follow up study of enhanced magnetic resonance imaging and clinical examination of the temporomandibular joint in children with juvenile idiopathic arthritis. *J. Rheumatol.* **2005**, *32*, 162–169. [PubMed]
66. Gozal, D.; Serpero, L.D.; Capdevila, O.; Kheirandish, S.; Gozal, L. Systemic inflammation in non-obese children with obstructive sleep apnea. *Sleep Med.* **2008**, *9*, 254–259. [CrossRef] [PubMed]
67. Marcus, C.L. Pathophysiology of childhood obstructive sleep apnea: Current concepts. *Respir. Physiol.* **2000**, *119*, 143–154. [CrossRef]
68. Ryan, D.P.O.; Bianchi, J.; Ignácio, J.; Wolford, L.M.; Gonçalves, J.R. Cone-beam computed tomography airway measurements: Can we trust them? *Am. J. Orthod. Dentofac. Orthop.* **2019**, *156*, 53–60. [CrossRef]
69. El, H.; Palomo, J.M. Measuring the airway in 3 dimensions: A reliability and accuracy study. *Am. J. Orthod. Dentofac. Orthop.* **2010**, *137* (Suppl. 4), S50.e1–S50.e9. [CrossRef]

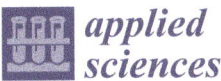

Article

Predictors of Analgesic Consumption in Orthodontic Patients

Jovana Juloski [1], Dina Vasovic [1,*], Ljiljana Vucic [1], Tina Pajevic [1], Nevena Gligoric [1], Mladen Mirkovic [2] and Branislav Glisic [1]

[1] Department of Orthodontics, School of Dental Medicine, University of Belgrade, Gastona Gravijea 2, 11000 Belgrade, Serbia; jovana.juloski@stomf.bg.ac.rs (J.J.); ljiljana.vucic@stomf.bg.ac.rs (L.V.); tina.pajevic@stomf.bg.ac.rs (T.P.); npuresevic@outlook.com (N.G.); branislav.glisic@stomf.bg.ac.rs (B.G.)
[2] Department of Orthodontics, Military Medical Academy, Crnotravska 17, 11000 Belgrade, Serbia; mladen.mirkovic@stomf.bg.ac.rs
* Correspondence: dina.vasovic@stomf.bg.ac.rs; Tel.: +381693702283

Abstract: During orthodontic treatment, pain is a subjective experience influenced by several factors. Orthodontic patients consume analgesics at different rates to alleviate this pain. Correlations between orthodontic pain and analgesic consumption were analyzed. Predictive factors to analgesics consumption were not statistically analyzed. This study was conducted to identify the predictive factors for analgesic consumption after initiation of orthodontic treatment with fixed appliances. Two hundred and eighty-six patients involved in this study kept a seven-day diary in which they recorded pain intensity (using a 0–10 numerical rating scale), analgesic consumption, localization of pain, pain triggers, and pain characteristics. Univariable analyses identified potential predictive factors: age, gender, pain intensity, pain localization, pain while chewing, pain at rest, night pain, headache, pulsating pain, sharp pain, dull pain, and tingling. Logistic regression was conducted to create a model that could predict analgesic consumption. Multivariate analyses demonstrated that analgesic consumption was increased by increased age, increased intensity of pain, and presence of a headache. Overall, the model explained 33% of analgesic requirement variability. Age, intensity of pain, and headache proved to be predictors of analgesic consumption. Knowledge of such factors may help clinicians identify orthodontic patients who will consume analgesics on their own.

Keywords: orthodontic pain; pain intensity; analgesics; VNS scale; buccal appliances; fixed orthodontic appliances; headache

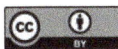

1. Introduction

During orthodontic treatment, after administration of orthodontic forces, patients experience pain. Orthodontic pain is a subjective experience influenced by several factors, such as patient's age, gender, orthodontic forces, emotional factors, type of orthodontic appliances, periodontal pain, bite forces, etc. [1–6]. Pain experienced in orthodontic patients treated with fixed orthodontic appliances is well established. It appears almost immediately after treatment initiation, peaks during the first day of treatment, and declines within the first week [7–9]. A certain percentage of patients still experience some pain after 7 days of treatment [7]. The intensity of orthodontic pain is mostly moderate, triggered by chewing and biting, and is usually described as discomfort or pressure [10]. In order to alleviate this pain orthodontic patients consume analgesics at different rates. According to relevant literature, about 30–40% of orthodontic patients consume self-administered analgesics [11,12]. Only correlations between orthodontic pain and analgesic consumption were analyzed [11].

To the best of our knowledge predictive factors to analgesics consumption, in order to alleviate orthodontic pain, were not statistically analyzed.

The aim of this study was to further analyze the predictors of analgesics consumption and to identify the predictive factors for self-administration of analgesics in orthodontic patients after initiation of orthodontic treatment with fixed appliances. The null hypothesis was that the intensity of pain is the only predictive factor for analgesic consumption.

2. Materials and Methods

The patients were enrolled consecutively in this trial which was performed at the University Orthodontic Department over the period of three years. For each patient, the treating orthodontic specialist made a treatment plan according to the patient's needs. The inclusion criteria for this investigation were: patients older than 11 years, healthy patients who have accepted necessary comprehensive orthodontic treatment with fixed buccal orthodontic appliances, patients that have signed informed consent. Exclusion criteria were patients consuming analgesics for other medical reasons, patients with cleft lip and/or palate, patients with syndromes, patients that were previously treated with fixed orthodontic appliances, and patients whose treatment included extra-oral appliances or additional intra-oral appliances (palatal arches, quad-helix, etc.).

For patients enrolled in the study, straight wire orthodontic appliances were bonded (brackets and tubes slot size 0.018", prescription Ricketts) with universal sealant and bonding primer (Ortho Solo by Ormco) and light cure orthodontic adhesive composite (Enlight by Ormco). All bonding appointments were scheduled between 9 a.m. and noon. After bonding, an initial superNiTi archwire was placed, whose size was assessed by the orthodontic specialist (0.012" or 0.014" depending on the degree of crowding). Immediately after bonding, all the patients included in the study were asked to keep a seven-day pain diary. At the beginning of the pain diary, the orthodontic specialist completed baseline data for each patient (age, gender, degree of crowding which was previously assessed on dental cast models, brackets prescription and slot size, archwire size, and tooth extractions prior to orthodontic treatment). All patients were verbally instructed to complete the pain diary at home, preferably each day at the same time, starting from 24 h after the orthodontic appointment until the seventh day. In the pain diaries, patients were asked to record their pain experience, by answering the questions concerning:

- pain initiation (with possible answers: immediately, after 6 h, after 12 h, it did not hurt), only for day 1,
- intensity of pain (reported on the Visual Numerical Scale (VNS), 0 to 10 scale, where 0 means no pain and 10 means extreme pain),
- analgesic consumption (with possible answers: yes and no),
- pain location (frontal teeth, posterior teeth, all teeth, it did not hurt),
- pain trigger (no pain, chewing, biting, cold food and drink, hot food and drink, at rest, during night, during physical activity),
- pain description (no pain, discomfort, pressure, tingling, dull pain, sharp pain, pulsating pain, headache).

All the questions in the pain diary were answered by circling one of the given answers, except for questions about pain triggers and description, where patients were allowed to circle each answer which coincided with their pain.

The analgesics were not prescribed by the orthodontic specialist. The patients were allowed to take analgesics as needed, and they recorded analgesic consumption for each day of the first week of treatment.

The pain diaries were collected from the patients on the following appointment.

Statistical Analysis

The data were analyzed to investigate differences between patients reporting analgesic consumption and those reporting no analgesics consumption during the first day of orthodontic treatment with fixed appliances. During the first day of orthodontic treatment 93 (33%) patients reported analgesic consumption (analgesics group), and 190 (67%) patients reported that they did not consume analgesics (no analgesics group).

Logistic regression (LR) analysis was used to test the investigated independent variables that would predict the need for analgesic consumption during the first day of the orthodontic treatment. Univariable analysis was performed to identify variables that would be included in the multivariate analysis. The forward and backward LR method was used in the multivariate analysis to create the preliminary model. The goodness-of-fit of the preliminary model was tested with the Hosmer–Lemeshow test. The results were presented as odds ratios with 95% confidence intervals. According to the sample size calculations, it was presumed that a sample of at least 220 patients should be enrolled in the study, keeping in mind that the sample size should be 10 times greater than the number of independent variables, which was 22 in this study. The sample size also proved to be sufficient in reference to the recommended rules of thumb formula EPV = 100 + 50 × i, where i refers to the number of independent variables in the final model, which was 3 in this study.

Statistical analysis was performed in IBM SPSS Statistics Data Editor (IBM SPSS version 21, Armonk, New York, NY, USA), with a level of statistical significance of $p < 0.05$.

3. Results

3.1. Sample Characteristics

Two hundred and eighty-six patients (90 males (31.5%), and 196 females (68.5%), aged 19.25 ± 6.60 years) involved in this study recorded that pain mostly started after 6 h (43%), followed by 12 h (35%) after the bonding procedure. The recorded intensity of pain for the first day after bonding was 4.03 ± 2.63 (median 4) (on VNS 1–10 scale), 3.763 ± 2.521 (median 4) for the second day, and 2.923 ± 2.309 (median 3) for the third day and continued to descend as the treatment progressed. Orthodontic patients consumed analgesics mostly during the first days of treatment, 33% of patients on the first day, 23% on the second day, about 9% on the third day. From the fourth day onward, less than 5% of patients consumed analgesics. Patients mostly complained that pain was triggered by chewing and biting, and described it as pressure and discomfort. In Table 1 the descriptive statistics of the investigated sample are given.

Table 1. Descriptive statistics for the investigated independent variables.

Parameter	Value	N	Percent	Mean (SD)	Median
Gender	Male	90	31.5		
	Female	196	68.5		
Age				19.25(6.60)	
Degree of crowding	Mild	107	45.5		
	Moderate	58	24.7		
	Severe	70	29.8		
Extraction therapy	Extraction	136	47.6		
	No extractions	150	52.4		
Wire size	0.012″	133	46.7		
	0.014″	140	49.1		
Beginning of pain	Immediately	19	6.7		
	After 6 h	123	43.2		
	After 12 h	99	34.7		
	Did not hurt	15	5.3		
Intensity of pain				4.03(2.63)	4
Pain killers	Yes	93	32.9		
	No	190	67.1		
Localization of the pain	Frontal teeth	105	36.8		
	Posterior teeth	46	16.1		
	All teeth	101	35.4		
	None	33	11.6		

Table 1. Cont.

Parameter	Value	N	Percent	Mean (SD)	Median
	Yes	26	9.1		
	No	260	90.9		
	Yes	190	66.4		
Pain triggers	No	95	33.2		
No pain	Yes	205	71.7		
Pain on bite	No	81	28.3		
Pain on chewing	Yes	11	3.8		
Pain on cold	No	274	95.8		
Pain on hot	Yes	8	2.8		
Pain at rest	No	278	97.2		
Pain at night	Yes	81	28.3		
Pain at physical activity	No	205	71.7		
	Yes	29	10.2		
	No	256	89.8		
	Yes	3	1.1		
	No	282	98.9		
	Yes	26	9.1		
	No	220	90.9		
	Yes	124	43.4		
Pain description	No	162	56.6		
No pain	Yes	175	61.2		
Discomfort	No	111	38.8		
Pressure	Yes	53	18.5		
Tingling	No	233	81.5		
Dull pain	Yes	74	25.9		
Sharp pain	No	212	74.1		
Pulsating pain	Yes	42	14.7		
Headache	No	244	85.3		
	Yes	47	16.5		
	No	237	83.5		
	Yes	30	10.5		
	No	256	89.5		

3.2. Predictors of Analgesic Consumption

Statistical analyses were performed for each of the possible predictive factors for analgesic consumption (age, gender, degree of crowding, archwire size, tooth extractions prior to orthodontic treatment, pain initiation, intensity of pain, pain location, chewing, biting, cold food and drink, hot food and drink, pain at rest, night pain, pain during physical activity, discomfort, pressure, tingling, dull pain, sharp pain, pulsating pain, and headache). In the first step, univariable analyses identified 12 potential predictive factors listed in Table 2.

Logistic regression was conducted to create a model that could predict analgesic consumption. The goodness-of-fit was tested with the Hosmer–Lemeshow test, the value of which signifies that the preliminary model was the final model. Multivariate analyses demonstrated that analgesic consumption was increased by increased age, increased intensity of pain, and presence of a headache, Table 3. With increasing age, for each year, the probability of the orthodontic patient consuming an analgesic in case of pain increases by 1.142, provided that the intensity of pain and the headache are controlled (remaining two factors). If the pain intensity increases, it also increases the probability that the patient will take an analgesic by 0.693, provided that the remaining factors are controlled. Orthodontic patients with headaches will take an analgesic 0.253 times more often than those who do not have a headache, provided that the other factors are controlled. Overall, the model explained 33% of analgesic requirement variability.

Table 2. Variables tested with univariable analysis whose *p* values were less than 0.25 and were therefore included in the further analysis.

Parameter		B	S.E.	Wald	df	p	OR	95% C.I.
Gender		0.670	0.290	5.335	1	0.021	1.955	1.107–3.454
Age		134	0.031	18.855	1	0.000	1.144	1.076–1.215
Intensity of pain		−0.392	0.059	44.072	1	0.000	0.676	0.602–0.758
Localization of the pain	Frontal	−1.624	0.640	6.435	1	0.011	0.197	0.056–0.691
	Posterior	−1.261	0.692	3.318	1	0.069	0.283	0.073–1.101
	All teeth	−2.038	0.639	10.190	1	0.001	0.130	0.037–0.455
	Constant	2.303	0.606	14.460	1	0.000	10.000	
Pain on chewing		−0.635	0.300	4.472	1	0.034	0.530	0.294–0.955
Pain at rest		−0.965	0.274	12.372	1	0.000	0.381	0.223–0.652
Pain at night		−0.739	0.396	3.487	1	0.062	0.478	0.220–1.037
Tingling		−0.502	0.315	2.546	1	0.111	0.605	0.326–1.122
Dull pain		−0.408	0.282	2.087	1	0.149	0.665	0.382–1.157
Sharp pain		−0.968	0.340	8.125	1	0.004	0.380	0.195–0.739
Pulsating pain		−1.256	0.329	14.552	1	0.000	0.285	0.149–0.543
Headache		−1.596	0.411	15.043	1	0.000	0.203	0.091–0.454

B—regression coefficient, S.E.—standard error, Wald—test value, df—degrees of freedom, OR—odds ratio, C.I—confidence interval.

Table 3. Parameters associated with analgesic consumption based on the final model of the logistic regression.

Parameter	B	S.E.	Wald	df	p	OR	95% C.I.
Age	0.133	0.035	14.184	1	0.000	1.142	1.066–1.224
Intensity of pain	−0.367	0.067	30.166	1	0.000	0.693	0.608–0.790
Headache	−1.376	0.494	7.760	1	0.005	0.253	0.096–0.665

Nagelkerke R^2 0.366, Hosmer–Lemeshow test 0.08.

4. Discussion

4.1. Summary of Main Findings

This investigation focused on analyzing the factors that could predict the need for analgesics consumption in orthodontic patients treated with fixed appliances. All the patients included in the study were divided into two groups—patients that consumed analgesics during the first day of orthodontic treatment and those who did not. Several variables were investigated: general characteristics, intensity of pain, pain location, pain triggers, and pain description. Our study has revealed that age, intensity of pain, and headaches proved to be predictors for analgesic consumption. The older the patients are, the higher the intensity of pain and if a headache is present, there is a higher chance that orthodontic patients will consume analgesics in order to alleviate pain caused by fixed orthodontic appliance treatment.

4.2. Predictors for Analgesic Consumption

Age, as one of the predictors for analgesic consumption, might be explained by the fact that as people get older, they are more used to controlling pain with analgesics, and less willing to put up with pain. The younger patients, besides the fact that they are not so used to controlling the pain with analgesics, are not able to take analgesics themselves, the analgesics have to be administered by their parents. Therefore, the observed difference in analgesic consumption between the patients of different ages. The literature is scarce regarding the topic of the present study. Regarding the association between the pain intensity and age, controversial results can be found [13–15]. In our study, both age and pain intensity were investigated separately, therefore the relationship between the intensity of pain and age would not have impacted the investigation.

The higher the intensity of pain, the more likely patients were to alleviate the pain with analgesics. Even though the average pain level on the first day of treatment of orthodontic patients was around 4, some of the patients experienced stronger pain. Almost 12% of patients reported a high pain level (8–10 on the VNS scale). Previous studies have also reported that analgesic intake correlated with pain intensity scores during orthodontic treatment [12,16]. This predictive factor was anticipated, therefore it was set as a null hypothesis.

Orthodontic pain sometimes reflects on the head, and patients report having headaches. This investigation reported that these patients are more likely to consume analgesics than patients without headaches if the two other factors are the same. In the present literature, the influence of headaches on analgesic consumption in orthodontic patients has not been investigated so far. The researchers have shown that the orthodontic pain pathway and headaches have related local inflammatory mechanisms transmitted by the trigeminal nerve, which may partially explain the presence of headaches in orthodontic patients [17]. Furthermore, the literature is ambiguous regarding the question of whether people with malocclusion were more likely to suffer from headaches [18].

It has been proved that peak pain intensity level is on the first day of orthodontic treatment [3,19,20]. The analgesics intake is correlated with pain intensity throughout the first week of orthodontic treatment [12]. These results are in concordance with the results in this study, therefore the data obtained for the first day of orthodontic treatment were used as representative. Analgesics consumption decreased significantly with each day of orthodontic treatment, reaching such low levels which could not be used for statistical analysis.

The pain caused by orthodontic treatment is sometimes underestimated, or even neglected. Patients treated with fixed orthodontic appliances experience pain and have the need to alleviate it with self-prescribed analgesics. The importance of analgesics consumption lies in the fact that there are implications that some analgesics could impact orthodontic tooth movement in terms of reducing it [21]. Monitoring of analgesics consumption has been proposed in order to avoid lengthening of treatment [21]. According to the results of the present study, attention can be also drawn to predictive factors (age, intensity of pain, and headaches). The results of this study indicate the need for further research on the association of orthodontic pain with the occurrence of a headache.

4.3. Limitations

Even though in this study, consumption of analgesics was investigated, not the characteristics of pain, investigating pain correlated features is difficult. The pain itself is a subjective feeling and has a broad range of interindividual differences [16,22–26] and therefore the analgesics consumption could be influenced. Furthermore, we should keep in mind that it was not possible to control completely the initial archwire size because of variations of patients' malocclusion and degree of initial crowding.

4.4. Strength

To the best of our knowledge, this is the first investigation on predictive factors for analgesic consumption in orthodontic patients. Different factors were analyzed as potential predictors, and three were confirmed to be predictors. In the present study, assessment of pain was performed daily, which is a more valid and reliable method, compared to retrospective response on recall [27].

5. Conclusions

Within the limitations of this study, the results revealed that age, intensity of pain, and headache are predictors for analgesic consumption.

Author Contributions: Conceptualization, J.J., D.V., L.V. and T.P.; methodology, J.J., D.V., N.G. and M.M.; software, J.J. and T.P.; formal analysis, T.P.; investigation, J.J., D.V., N.G. and M.M.; resources, J.J., D.V., L.V., N.G. and T.P.; data curation, J.J., D.V., L.V., T.P. and N.G.; writing—original draft preparation, J.J., D.V., L.V., T.P. and N.G.; writing—review and editing, B.G.; supervision, B.G. All authors have read and agreed to the published version of the manuscript.

Funding: This research received no external funding.

Institutional Review Board Statement: The Institutional Ethical Board of School of Dentistry University of Belgrade, Serbia (No 36/15) has approved the protocol for this clinical trial.

Informed Consent Statement: Informed consent was obtained from all subjects involved in the study. Written informed consent was obtained from the patient(s) or parent/legal guardian to publish this paper.

Data Availability Statement: Not applicable.

Conflicts of Interest: The authors declare no conflict of interest.

References

1. Sergl, H.G.; Klages, U.; Zentner, A. Pain and discomfort during orthodontic treatment: Causative factors and effects on compliance. *Am. J. Orthod. Dentofac. Orthop.* **1998**, *114*, 684–691. [CrossRef]
2. Sergl, H.G.; Zentner, A. A comparative assessment of acceptance of different types of functional appliances. *Eur. J. Orthod.* **1998**, *20*, 517–524. [CrossRef] [PubMed]
3. Curto, A.; Albaladejo, A.; Montero, J.; Alvarado-Lorenzo, M.; Garcovich, D.; Alvarado-Lorenzo, A. A Prospective Randomized Clinical Trial to Evaluate the Slot Size on Pain and Oral Health-Related Quality of Life (OHRQoL) in Orthodontics during the First Month of Treatment with Conventional and Low-Friction Brackets. *Appl. Sci.* **2020**, *10*, 7136. [CrossRef]
4. Alcón, S.; Curto, A.; Alvarado, M.; Albaladejo, A.; Garcovich, D.; Alvarado-Lorenzo, A. Comparative Analysis of Periodontal Pain Using Two Different Orthodontic Techniques, Fixed Multibrackets and Removable Aligners: A Longitudinal Clinical Study with Monthly Follow-Ups for 12 Months. *Appl. Sci.* **2021**, *11*, 12013. [CrossRef]
5. Alam, M.K.; Ganji, K.K.; Meshari, A.; Manay, S.M.; Bin Jamayet, N.; Siddiqui, A.A. Pain Management Using Nano-Bio Fusion Gel in Fixed Orthodontic Therapy-Induced Gingivitis: A Split-Mouth Design Study. *Appl. Sci.* **2021**, *11*, 11463. [CrossRef]
6. Therkildsen, N.M.; Sonnesen, L. Bite Force, Occlusal Contact and Pain in Orthodontic Patients during Fixed-Appliance Treatment. *Dent. J.* **2022**, *10*, 14. [CrossRef]
7. Scheurer, P.A.; Firestone, A.R.; Bürgin, W.B. Perception of pain as a result of orthodontic treatment with fixed appliances. *Eur. J. Orthod.* **1996**, *18*, 349–357. [CrossRef]
8. Ngan, P.; Kess, B.; Wilson, S. Perception of discomfort by patients undergoing orthodontic treatment. *Am. J. Orthod. Dentofac. Orthop.* **1989**, *96*, 47–53. [CrossRef]
9. Wiedel, A.-P.; Bondemark, L. A randomized controlled trial of self-perceived pain, discomfort, and impairment of jaw function in children undergoing orthodontic treatment with fixed or removable appliances. *Angle Orthod.* **2016**, *86*, 324–330. [CrossRef]
10. Markovic, E.; Fercec, J.; Scepan, I.; Glisic, B.; Nedeljkovic, N.; Juloski, J.; Rudolf, R. The correlation between pain perception among patients with six different orthodontic archwires and the degree of dental crowding. *Srp. Arh. Celok. Lek.* **2015**, *143*, 134–140. [CrossRef]
11. Juloski, J.; Vasović, D.; Vučić, L.; Pajević, T.; Glišić, B. Orthodontic pain in maxilla and mandible during the first week of orthodontic treatment. *Balk. J. Dent. Med.* **2022**, *26*, 33–40. [CrossRef]
12. Miller, K.B.; McGorray, S.P.; Womack, R.; Quintero, J.C.; Perelmuter, M.; Gibson, J.; Dolan, T.A.; Wheeler, T.T. A comparison of treatment impacts between Invisalign aligner and fixed appliance therapy during the first week of treatment. *Am. J. Orthod. Dentofac. Orthop.* **2007**, *131*, 302.e1–302.e9. [CrossRef] [PubMed]
13. da Costa, E.O.; Blagitz, M.N.; Normando, D. Impact of catastrophizing on pain during orthodontic treatment. *Dent. Press J. Orthod.* **2020**, *25*, 64–69. [CrossRef] [PubMed]
14. Brown, D.F.; Moerenhout, R.G. The pain experience and psychological adjustment to orthodontic treatment of preadolescents, adolescents, and adults. *Am. J. Orthod. Dentofac. Orthop.* **1991**, *100*, 349–356. [CrossRef]
15. Abdelrahman, R.S.; Al-Nimri, K.S.; Al Maaitah, E.F. Pain experience during initial alignment with three types of nickel-titanium archwires: A prospective clinical trial. *Angle Orthod.* **2015**, *85*, 1021–1026. [CrossRef]
16. Erdinç, A.M.E.; Dinçer, B. Perception of pain during orthodontic treatment with fixed appliances. *Eur. J. Orthod.* **2004**, *26*, 79–85. [CrossRef]
17. Tang, Z.; Zhou, J.; Long, H.; Gao, Y.; Wang, Q.; Li, X.; Wang, Y.; Lai, W.; Jian, F. Molecular mechanism in trigeminal nerve and treatment methods related to orthodontic pain. *J. Oral Rehabil.* **2022**, *49*, 125–137. [CrossRef]
18. Komazaki, Y.; Fujiwara, T.; Ogawa, T.; Sato, M.; Suzuki, K.; Yamagata, Z.; Moriyama, K. Association between malocclusion and headache among 12- to 15-year-old adolescents: A population-based study. *Community Dent. Oral Epidemiol.* **2014**, *42*, 572–580. [CrossRef]
19. Sandhu, S.S.; Leckie, G. Diurnal variation in orthodontic pain: Clinical implications and pharmacological management. *Semin. Orthod.* **2018**, *24*, 217–224. [CrossRef]
20. Cozzani, M.; Ragazzini, G.; Delucchi, A.; Barreca, C.; Rinchuse, D.J.; Servetto, R.; Calevo, M.G.; Piras, V. Self-reported pain after orthodontic treatments: A randomized controlled study on the effects of two follow-up procedures. *Eur. J. Orthod.* **2016**, *38*, 266–271. [CrossRef]

21. Haas, D.A. An update on analgesics for the management of acute postoperative dental pain. *J.-Can. Dent. Assoc.* **2002**, *68*, 476–484. [PubMed]
22. Bergius, M.; Berggren, U.; Kiliaridis, S. Experience of pain during an orthodontic procedure. *Eur. J. Oral Sci.* **2002**, *110*, 92–98. [CrossRef] [PubMed]
23. Bergius, M.; Kiliaridis, S.; Berggren, U. Pain in orthodontics. *J. Orofac. Orthop./Fortschr. Kieferorthopädie* **2000**, *61*, 125–137. [CrossRef] [PubMed]
24. Krishnan, V. Orthodontic pain: From causes to management—A review. *Eur. J. Orthod.* **2007**, *29*, 170–179. [CrossRef]
25. Krukemeyer, A.M.; Arruda, A.O.; Inglehart, M.R. Pain and Orthodontic Treatment: Patient Experiences and Provider Assessments. *Angle Orthod.* **2009**, *79*, 1175–1181. [CrossRef] [PubMed]
26. Xiaoting, L.; Yin, T.; Yangxi, C. Interventions for pain during fixed orthodontic appliance therapy. A systematic review. *Angle Orthod.* **2010**, *80*, 925–932. [CrossRef]
27. Carp, F.M.; Carp, A. The validity, reliability and generalizability of diary data. *Exp. Aging Res.* **1981**, *7*, 281–296. [CrossRef]

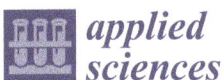

Article

Gingival Recessions and Periodontal Status after Minimum 2-Year-Retention Post-Non-Extraction Orthodontic Treatment

Livia Nastri [1], Ludovica Nucci [2], Domenico Carozza [2], Stefano Martina [3], Ismene Serino [4], Letizia Perillo [2], Fabrizia d'Apuzzo [2,*] and Vincenzo Grassia [2]

1 Periodontal Unit, Multidisciplinary Department of Medical-Surgical and Dental Specialties, University of Campania Luigi Vanvitelli, 80138 Naples, Italy; livia.nastri@unicampania.it
2 Orthodontic Program, Multidisciplinary Department of Medical-Surgical and Dental Specialties, University of Campania Luigi Vanvitelli, 80138 Naples, Italy; ludovica.nucci@unicampania.it (L.N.); domicarozza1@gmail.com (D.C.); letizia.perillo@unicampania.it (L.P.); grassiavincenzo@libero.it (V.G.)
3 Department of Medicine, Surgery and Dentistry "Scuola Medica Salernitana", University of Salerno, 84081 Baronissi, Italy; smartina@unisa.it
4 Department of Experimental Medicine, University of Campania Luigi Vanvitelli, 80138 Naples, Italy; ismene.serino@unicampania.it
* Correspondence: fabrizia.dapuzzo@unicampania.it; Tel.: +39-081-566-5495 or +39-338-482-0462

Citation: Nastri, L.; Nucci, L.; Carozza, D.; Martina, S.; Serino, I.; Perillo, L.; d'Apuzzo, F.; Grassia, V. Gingival Recessions and Periodontal Status after Minimum 2-Year-Retention Post-Non-Extraction Orthodontic Treatment. *Appl. Sci.* **2022**, *12*, 1641. https://doi.org/10.3390/app12031641

Academic Editor: Bruno Chrcanovic

Received: 13 January 2022
Accepted: 2 February 2022
Published: 4 February 2022

Publisher's Note: MDPI stays neutral with regard to jurisdictional claims in published maps and institutional affiliations.

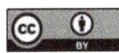

Copyright: © 2022 by the authors. Licensee MDPI, Basel, Switzerland. This article is an open access article distributed under the terms and conditions of the Creative Commons Attribution (CC BY) license (https://creativecommons.org/licenses/by/4.0/).

Abstract: The objectives of this study were to assess gingival recessions (GR) and periodontal status in patients previously treated with non-extraction orthodontic treatment and retention at a follow-up of a minimum of two years after the end of treatment. Data from patients aged between 16 and 35 years with a previous non-extraction orthodontic treatment and at least 2 years of retention and full records before and after treatment were collected. The casts were digitalized using the 3Shape TRIOS® intraoral scanner and the Viewbox4 software was used for the measurements. The following parameters were scored: inclination of the lower and upper incisors (IMPA and I^SN) and anterior crowding (Little index). The included patients were recalled for a clinical periodontal follow-up examination and the following parameters were evaluated: buccal and lingual GR (mm) of incisors and canines, bleeding of probing score, plaque score, and gingival phenotype. The digital cast analysis showed a mean Little index of 7.78 (SD 5.83) and 1.39 (SD 0.79), respectively, before and after treatment. The initial and final cephalometric analyses showed an I^SN of 103.53° and 105.78° (SD 7.21) and IMPA of 91.3° and 95.1°, respectively. At the follow-up periodontal visits, the patients showed an overall low oral hygiene with bleeding at probing in 66.6% and plaque in the anterior area in 76.2% of patients. From the total examined 240 teeth of the frontal sextants, three patients had GR (from 1 to 6.5 mm): in the upper arch two at canines and one at central incisor, whereas in the lower arch two at central and one at lateral incisors. The gingival phenotype was thick in 55% of cases. The lingual-to-lingual retainers at follow-up were present in 61.9% of patients. A slight increased risk for buccal GR development was found only in correlation with the presence of fixed retainer and thin gingival phenotype mainly in patients with gingivitis. Thus, non-extraction orthodontic treatment performed with controlled forces and biomechanics seems to not affect the development of GR or the periodontal health after retention.

Keywords: gingival recessions; periodontal status; orthodontic treatment; retention; digital casts

1. Introduction

Gingival recession (GR) is defined as the apical shift of the gingival margin with respect to the cementoenamel junction (CEJ) [1]; it is associated with attachment loss and exposure of the root surface to the oral environment [2–4]. GR may cause pain, increased tooth sensitivity, compromised aesthetics, and the onset of carious/noncarious cervical lesions (NCCL). Romandini et al. [5] have reported that over 90% of the adult population in the United States have mid-buccal–gingival recessions whose 70% is in the aesthetic zone.

In a subpopulation of subjects from 30 to 39 years of age, the prevalence of GR was assessed as 37.8% mainly on the buccal sites of the teeth [6]. Several predisposing risk factors have been suggested, such as periodontal phenotype, tooth type and position in the dental arch, amount of attached gingiva, and lack of alveolar buccal bone as well as age, gender, and ethnicity [7–13]. In particular, a thin gingival phenotype was described as a risk factor for inflammation-related GR in the presence of tooth-brushing trauma [14,15] and poor oral hygiene with plaque accumulation [16].

Other studies have also reported that the application of orthodontic forces in specific direction of tooth movements could increase the development or progression of GR during treatment or later in the retention phase [16–19]. According to a recent consensus report on the classification of periodontal and peri-implant diseases and conditions [20], soft tissue alteration can be associated with the buccal–lingual thickness of the gingiva and to the application of orthodontic forces moving teeth out of the alveolar envelope with a localized bony dehiscence and fenestrations [21–23]. A higher prevalence or severity of GR both during and after orthodontic treatment was specifically detected after excessive mandibular incisor proclination [24–27].

Conversely, other authors did not find significant differences in prevalence or severity of GR in orthodontically treated patients compared to a matched non-treated sample [28–32], but other factors such as adulthood and the amount of keratinized gingiva were considered relevant in the onset of GR despite the orthodontic technique applied [33]. Thus, the available literature on this topic is still highly debated and three systematic reviews have summarized the main outcomes [16,19,24]. Joss Vassalli et al. [16] confirmed that an excessive incisor movement out of the bone alveolar process could be associated with a higher tendency for developing GR and more buccally proclined teeth had a higher severity of it. However, the same authors commented that the clinical significance of this GR amount may be questionable. Tepedino et al. [34] included only two studies after the qualitative analysis and reported that the effects of orthodontic treatment on the development of GR were not statistically or clinically significant. Therefore, these findings demonstrated weak evidence due to short-term follow up and a significant number of confounding variables without control of the heterogeneity in outcome assessment among the studies, not allowing an adequate meta-analysis. A more recent systematic review of Bin Bahar et al. [19], including three papers with a quantitative analysis on two of them, concluded that an increased risk for GR development on the anterior teeth could be encountered in orthodontically treated compared to untreated individuals with normal occlusion, especially during retention, although the amount of GR did not significantly differ in the whole sample. In conclusion, this topic is highly debated and evidence-based data are still not available on gingival status in orthodontic patients after the retention phase compared to treatment outcomes after non-extraction treatment with fixed appliances.

Thus, the aim of this study was to assess GR and periodontal status in a group of patients previously treated with non-extraction orthodontic treatments and retention with a follow up of minimum two years after the end of active treatment.

2. Materials and Methods

The research protocol of this observational study was approved by the Ethics Committee of the University of Campania *Luigi Vanvitelli* (Prot. n°18/2018) and a signed informed consent for the use of personal data was available. Data recruitment started in March 2020 and the sample included patients who had consecutively completed their orthodontic treatment between October 2012 and February 2018 at the Orthodontic Program of the University of Campania *Luigi Vanvitelli*, Naples (Italy). The inclusion criteria were an age between 17 and 35 years; a two-phase non-extraction orthodontic treatment (except for the third molars) with fixed appliances completed at least two years before data collection; the presence of all six dental elements of the frontal upper and lower sextant; and initial and final orthodontic records (lateral cephalometrics, intra/oral photographs, and dental casts of good quality) (Figure 1). The exclusion criteria were systemic pathologies or intake of drugs affecting the periodontal status; periodontitis and/or gingival recessions before the beginning of the orthodontic treatment; and the presence of labial or lingual piercings.

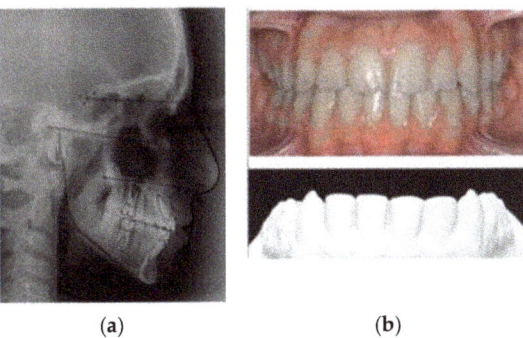

(a)   (b)

Figure 1. Post-orthodontic treatment records: cephalometrics (a), photographs, and dental casts (b).

The orthodontic treatment performed in all cases involved in this study included maxillary expander and/or transpalatal arch in the upper and lip bumper in the lower arch during mixed dentition followed by multibracket fixed appliances (MBT prescription) and retention at the end of treatment.

The dental casts were digitalized using the TRIOS® 3Shape intraoral scanner. The Viewbox 4 software (dHal Software, Kifissia, Greece) was used for the measurements on digital models and cephalograms by the same trained operator and the following values were evaluated:

- Anterior crowding through the Little's irregularity index, defined as the sum of displacement of the anatomic contact points of the mandibular anterior teeth [35];
- Inclination of the lower incisors to the mandibular plane (IMPA) and of the upper incisors to the sellar plane (I^SN).

The gingival phenotype was clinically evaluated on the general appearance of the gingiva around the tooth and probing the sulcus: the gingival phenotype was considered thin if the gingiva were delicate, friable, and almost translucent and the periodontal probe were visible through the gingival tissue, whereas it was considered thick if the gingiva were dense and fibrotic in appearance and the probe were not visible [36].

At the clinical recall appointment, a questionnaire on general health and oral hygiene habits (type and frequency of toothbrushing, interdental cleaning, oral washes use) was delivered to each included patient.

A periodontist evaluated the periodontal status and assessed the following parameters:

- Gingival recession, measured in mm as the distance between the CEJ and coronal margin of the free gingiva, approximated to the nearest 0.5 mm, both on the buccal and lingual surfaces of teeth in the II and V sextants;
- Probing pocket depth (PPD), measured with the Williams-Goldman periodontal probe as the distance from the free gingival margin to the bottom of the sulcus/pocket and approximated to the nearest millimeter at 6 points for each tooth in the II and V sextants;
- Gingival inflammation, evaluated with the Bleeding On Probing (BOP) score according to Ainamo and Bay [37];
- Presence of plaque, evaluated with the Plaque Control record (O'Leary) [38] for the II and V sextants.

If calculus or plaque were present on the tooth surfaces, it was removed before measuring the gingival recessions. The presence and type of orthodontic retention and the evaluation of its integrity were checked during the same appointment by an orthodontist.

Statistical Analysis

On the data collected, a descriptive statistical analysis was performed with calculation of the mean and standard deviation. The odds ratio (OR) was used as the risk ratio of association between an exposure and an outcome and represents the odds that an outcome will occur given a particular exposure, compared to the odds of the outcome occurring in the absence of that exposure. Data analysis was performed using the SSPS software. The significance was set at a p value < 0.05.

3. Results

Sixty-three patients met the inclusion criteria and were recalled for follow-up periodontal and orthodontic examinations. Out of these, 22 patients did not respond, or their telephone number was not active while 10 were transferred out of the country and refused to come. These patients were examined at the Orthodontic and Periodontal Programs of the University of Campania Luigi Vanvitelli. They were first interviewed about their current general anamnesis (diabetes, hypertension, endocrine diseases, disvitaminosis, dysmetabolism, heart diseases, kidney diseases, state of nutrition, pregnancy, allergy, ongoing pharmacological therapies), and the presence of all anterior upper and lower dental elements was evaluated. After these follow-up analyses, further 11 patients were excluded.

Thus, a final sample of 20 subjects (9 males and 11 female) ranged between 17.1 and 31.10 years (mean age 11.9 ± 3.7 years) proceeded with complete periodontal clinical examination. Of these patients, orthodontic and clinical records (dental casts, lateral radiographs and clinical charts) before (T0) and at the end of the active orthodontic fixed treatment (T1) were examined (Table 1).

Table 1. Sample sizes and ages (y), at T0 (the start of orthodontic treatment), T1 (the end of orthodontic treatment), and T2 (follow-up) for the overall sample and subgroups.

Group	Subgroup	n	T0		T1		Mean tx Time		T2	
			Mean	SD	Mean	SD	Mean	SD	Mean	SD
Overall		20	11.9	3.7	16.2	3.1	4.4	1.8	21.0	3.2
Sex	Male	9	10.8	1.6	15.4	1.8			20.8	1.9
	Female	11	12.9	4.6	17.0	3.8			21.1	3.9

The recruited patients started with the following Angle dental class of malocclusion: 7 patients with Class I, 11 patients with Class II (of which 2 with Class II, division 2), 2 patients with Class III and they were orthodontically treated without tooth extraction (except third molars) with a first phase including maxillary expander and/or transpalatal arch followed by fixed multibrackets appliances in permanent dentition all achieving a Class I. The average treatment duration was of 4.4 years (SD 1.8) (Table 1).

The digital cast analysis before (T0) and at the end (T1) of the orthodontic treatment reported a mean Little's index of 6.83 (SD 3.41) and 1.79 (SD 1.49), respectively (Table 2).

Table 2. Digital cast and cephalometric analysis before (T0) and at the end (T1) of the orthodontic treatment.

	T0		T1		ΔT1−T0		p
	Mean	SD	Mean	SD	Mean	SD	
Little index (mm)	6.83	3.41	1.79	1.49	5.04	3.44	0.001 *
I^SN (°)	103.50	7.11	106.20	8.07	2.70	11.37	0.268
IMPA (°)	91.4	7.4	95.1	10.3	3.625	8.13	0.206

* $p < 0.05$.

The relationship between Little's index at T0 and the GR development was not present (Table 3). The initial and final cephalometric analyses showed an I^SN angle of 103.50° (SD 7.11) and 106.20° (SD 8.07), and an IMPA of 91.4° (SD 7.4) and 95.1° (SD 10.3), respectively (Table 2). No correlation was shown between incisors inclination and GR (Table 3).

Table 3. Little irregularity index and GR.

Little Index (mm) from 1–3	GR Yes	GR No	from 3–6	GR Yes	GR No	from 6–9	GR Yes	GR No
exposed	1	5		1	8		1	7
non-exposed	2	12		2	9		2	10
OR: 1.201				OR: 0.444			OR: 0.714	

About the periodontal follow-up recall, from the 240 teeth of the frontal sextants (II and V sextant) examined, 6 teeth had GR (ranging from 1 to 6.5 mm), found in three patients. A total of three of these were present in the upper arch and three in the lower arch. In the upper arch two GR were located on the canines, one was on a central incisor, while in the lower arch, all recessions were present on incisors (one central and one lateral).

Only 2.5% of the total teeth showed buccal GR, and significant results were detected with the odds ratio calculation. From the periodontal point of view, at the beginning of the orthodontic treatment, patients of our sample had a slight prevalence of thick gingival phenotype (n°11) compared to thin phenotype (n°9). An odds ratio of 2.857 for the thin phenotype was reported in association to buccal GR, indicating a tendency to be a risk factor. The lingual-to-lingual lower retainers at follow-up were present in the 61.9% of patients while the others wore removable appliances. A good association was shown between fixed retainers and GR development with an odds ratio of 2,857 (Table 4).

Table 4. Incisor inclinations, gingival phenotype, fixed retainer and GR.

I^SN > 102°	GR Yes	GR No	IMPA > 95°	GR Yes	GR No	Gingival Phenotype	GR Yes	GR No	Fixed Retainer	GR Yes	GR No
exposed	2	10		1	6	thin	2	7	present	2	7
non-exposed	1	7		2	11	thick	1	10	absent	1	10
OR: 0.350			OR: 0.917			OR: 2.857			OR: 2.857		

Most patients reported brushing twice a day with a manual toothbrush, without the use of dental floss. The use of a reduced brushing frequency (no more than 2 times per day) associated with the lack of cleansing of the interdental spaces may be partly responsible for the observation of increased plaque and bleeding (Table 5). The periodontal biometric parameters did not result in any correlation with GR, neither if analyzed on a patient basis, nor if analyzed on an arch basis or single site. Thus, there was no clear correlation between GR and brushing type and frequency (Table 5).

Table 5. Anamnestic data at follow-up.

Gingival Phenotype		Brushing Frequency		Interdental Cleaning			Mouthwash		
Thick	Thin	2/Day	3/Day	No	Floss	Brush	Occasionally	2/Day	No
11	9	15	5	16	2	1	6	4	10

At the time of observation for the present study, the periodontal conditions were characterized by the presence of a mean plaque index in sextant II of 20.69% (SD 31.74%) and a mean plaque index in sextant V of 45.42% (SD 37.88%). Only 6 of 20 patients had an overall plaque index <20%. Bleeding on probing was 19.17% (SD 16.37%) in sextant II and 40.28% (SD 25.18%) in sextant V, with a similar trend, as expected, with respect to the presence of bacterial plaque. Only five patients had <20% bleeding in both sextants analyzed. The mean probing depth for sextant V was 2.08 (SD 0.38), while the corresponding value for sextant II was 2.04 (SD 0.41) (Table 6). Only one of the patients had pathological probing depths >3 mm in almost all of the sites of the two sextants analyzed.

Table 6. Periodontal parameters at follow-up.

	Upper Arch		Lower Arch		Full Arch	
	Mean	SD	Mean	SD	Mean	SD
PPD (mm)	2.04	0.41	2.08	0.38	2.06	0.39
BOP (%)	19.17%	16.37%	40.28%	25.18%	29.72%	23.53%
plaque presence (%)	20.69%	31.74%	45.42%	37.88%	33.06%	36.69%

4. Discussion

Orthodontic treatment is frequently an elective procedure performed mostly for aesthetic reasons. GR and periodontal diseases may compromise the smile esthetics and general oral health. According to the literature, the prevalence in the general population of GR, mainly buccal, is high tending to increase with age, and sites with recessions were susceptible for additional apical displacement and loss of periodontal support [39]. The aim of this investigation was to recruit only patients without any recession at the start of the orthodontic treatment in order to identify the role of orthodontic treatment in GR occurrence at minimum 2-yr of follow-up. The outcomes of our study showed a very low prevalence of GR compared to the epidemiologic value in the general population at the same age. However, our sample, collected with strict exclusion criteria, showed a prevalence of GR in only 2.5% of teeth included in our post-retention clinical examination. This was in accordance with the prevalence and distribution found in a cross-sectional and longitudinal study showing a very low occurrence of GR after a follow-up of 12 years of observation in non-treated patients who did not show recessions at baseline [39]. Gebistorf et al. [30] also evaluated recessions after the retention phase in a population of 88 subjects. However, the prevalence of recessions at baseline was 55%, thus justifying the value of 98.9% at post-retention examination. GR has many confounding predisposing and etiological factors. Orthodontic treatment is one of the more debated iatrogenic factors that have been implicated in its occurrence. According to Sawan et al. [33], non-extraction treatment is related to an increase in risk, with the intercanine width as a negative predictor of gingival recessions. In this study inclination of the incisors was not statistically significant to GR. This in accordance with Morris et al. [31] who found no correlation with incisor proclination (IMPA > 95°) in a post-retention population. In our study we did not find any correlation between GR and final IMPA value, even when this value was higher than 95°, nor with the change of inclination. The change of inclination has been claimed as a factor responsible for the occurrence of GR. According to Pernet et al. [26] patients with buccal or lingual recessions presented a mean incisor inclination change of 3° (range: −9° to 23°); however, the authors found that among the patients with a more than 10° inclination change, 12 out of 16 had no recessions. Comparing the prevalence observed in our study, the outcome is similar to Renkema et al. [27] looking at their 2 years of observation. In their study GR increased after 5 years of treatment, but this difference can be confounded by the increase in age of the sample. Although the prevalence of recessions in our study is lower, this could be due to a shorter observation time in our investigation.

According to Vasconcelos et al. [28], incisor retroclination was more correlated to GR than proclination of lower incisors, even if the buccal positioning of central incisors are indicated as a major risk factor for its development. Their results indicated a low prevalence of GR after orthodontic treatment, in accordance with our observation, but did not indicate gingival phenotype as a risk factor as well as gingival inflammation, that was found in 29.72 ± 23.53% of the examined teeth without correlation to GR. Visible plaque and calculus were a frequent observation (33.06 ± 36.03%). Pandis et al. [40] argue that the presence of a fixed retainer increased the calculus, which possibly contributed to the increase in the number of lingual recessions. However, the presence of the bonded retainer was not correlated with gingivitis or with recessions, all of them found labially. Our findings do not confirm a correlation between bonded retainer and gingivitis or recessions. The overall adherence to oral hygiene effective measures of interdental cleaning was low in our sample, and this can justify the observed high level of plaque and gingivitis. GR may occur as a consequence of alveolar dehiscence, and it seems crucial to apply light forces on multiple teeth rather than to a single tooth [41]. Moreover, discrepancies such as the low prevalence of GR in our study can also be explained by differences in age at assessment, methods of evaluation, or various behavioral influences (hygiene, smoking, and professional periodontal treatment) compared to previous evaluations [5]. The odds ratio was used in this study to approximate the risk ratio because the prevalence of the GR was low, and it an association was detected with the presence of lower fixed retainer and thin phenotype, confirming previous findings [16].

The limitations of this study are the small sample size and the retrospective nature of clinical records before and at the end of the orthodontic treatment, thus the outcomes do not allow definitive statements. Further studies, including a longer follow-up of patients with the similar dentoskeletal characteristics and further prospective assessment of gingival crevicular fluid in patients during and after orthodontic treatment using new and reliable techniques [42], may help to investigate the reasons for GR occurrence in adults and orthodontic population.

5. Conclusions

Based on the findings and within the limitations of this study, a non-extraction orthodontic treatment seems to not affect either the development of buccal or lingual recessions or the periodontal status after at least two years of retention post-orthodontics. A slight increased risk for buccal GR development was found only in correlation with the presence of fixed retainer and thin gingival phenotype mainly in patients with gingivitis. Thus, periodical periodontal follow-up appointments after orthodontic treatment are needed to motivate subjects in maintaining a better oral hygiene in the adulthood.

Author Contributions: Conceptualization, L.P. and L.N. (Livia Nastri); methodology, F.d., I.S. and V.G.; data curation, L.N. (Livia Nastri) and L.N. (Ludovica Nucci); writing—original draft preparation, L.N. (Ludovica Nucci) and F.d.; writing—review and editing, S.M. and D.C.; supervision, L.P. and V.G. All authors have read and agreed to the published version of the manuscript.

Funding: This research received no external funding.

Institutional Review Board Statement: The study was conducted in accordance with the Declaration of Helsinki and approved by the Institutional Review Board of the University of Campania *Luigi Vanvitelli* (protocol code n°18/2018).

Informed Consent Statement: Informed consent was obtained from all subjects involved in the study.

Data Availability Statement: The data presented in this study are available on request from the corresponding author. The data are not publicly available due to privacy restrictions.

Conflicts of Interest: The authors declare no conflict of interest.

Abbreviations

GR	gingival recession
CEJ	cemento-enamel junction
NCCL	noncarious cervical lesions
IMPA	inclination of the lower incisors to the mandibular plane
I^SN	upper incisors to the sellar plane
PPD	probing pocket depth
BOP	bleeding on probing

References

1. Pini Prato, G. Mucogingival Deformities. *Ann. Periodontol.* **1999**, *4*, 98–101. [CrossRef]
2. Cortellini, P.; Bissada, N.F. Mucogingival Conditions in the Natural Dentition: Narrative Review, Case Definitions, and Diagnostic Considerations. *J. Clin. Periodontol.* **2018**, *45* (Suppl. 2), S190–S198. [CrossRef] [PubMed]
3. Renkema, A.M.; Fudalej, P.S.; Renkema, A.A.P.; Abbas, F.; Bronkhorst, E.; Katsaros, C. Gingival Labial Recessions in Orthodontically Treated and Untreated Individuals: A Case—Control Study. *J. Clin. Periodontol.* **2013**, *40*, 631–637. [CrossRef] [PubMed]
4. Zucchelli, G.; Mounssif, I. Periodontal Plastic Surgery. *Periodontol. 2000* **2015**, *68*, 333–368. [CrossRef] [PubMed]
5. Romandini, M.; Soldini, M.C.; Montero, E.; Sanz, M. Epidemiology of Mid-Buccal Gingival Recessions in NHANES According to the 2018 World Workshop Classification System. *J. Clin. Periodontol.* **2020**, *47*, 1180–1190. [CrossRef]
6. Albandar, J.M.; Kingman, A. Gingival Recession, Gingival Bleeding, and Dental Calculus in Adults 30 Years of Age and Older in the United States, 1988–1994. *J. Periodontol.* **1999**, *70*, 30–43. [CrossRef]
7. Hudecki, A.; Kiryczyński, G.; Łos, M.J. Biomaterials, Definition, Overview. In *Stem Cells and Biomaterials for Regenerative Medicine*; Łos, M.J., Hudecki, A., Wiecheć, E., Eds.; Elsevier: Amsterdam, The Netherlands, 2019.
8. Holtfreter, B.; Schwahn, C.; Biffar, R.; Kocher, T. Epidemiology of Periodontal Diseases in the Study of Health in Pomerania. *J. Clin. Periodontol.* **2009**, *36*, 114–123. [CrossRef]
9. Löe, H.; Anerud, A.; Boysen, H. The Natural History of Periodontal Disease in Man: Prevalence, Severity, and Extent of Gingival Recession. *J. Periodontol.* **1992**, *63*, 489–495. [CrossRef]
10. Rios, F.S.; Costa, R.S.A.; Moura, M.S.; Jardim, J.J.; Maltz, M.; Haas, A.N. Estimates and Multivariable Risk Assessment of Gingival Recession in the Population of Adults from Porto Alegre, Brazil. *J. Clin. Periodontol.* **2014**, *41*, 1098–1107. [CrossRef]
11. Sarfati, A.; Bourgeois, D.; Katsahian, S.; Mora, F.; Bouchard, P. Risk Assessment for Buccal Gingival Recession Defects in an Adult Population. *J. Periodontol.* **2010**, *81*, 1419–1425. [CrossRef]
12. Susin, C.; Haas, A.N.; Oppermann, R.V.; Haugejorden, O.; Albandar, J.M. Gingival Recession: Epidemiology and Risk Indicators in a Representative Urban Brazilian Population. *J. Periodontol.* **2004**, *75*, 1377–1386. [CrossRef]
13. Zucchelli, G.; Mounssif, I.; Marzadori, M.; Mazzotti, C.; Felice, P.; Stefanini, M. Connective Tissue Graft Wall Technique and Enamel Matrix Derivative for the Treatment of Infrabony Defects: Case Reports. *Int. J. Periodontics Restor. Dent.* **2017**, *37*, 673–681. [CrossRef] [PubMed]
14. Agudio, G.; Cortellini, P.; Buti, J.; Pini Prato, G. Periodontal conditions of sites treated with gingival augmentation surgery compared with untreated contralateral homologous sites: An 18- to 35-year long-term study. *J. Periodontol.* **2016**, *87*, 1371–1378. [CrossRef] [PubMed]
15. Chambrone, L.; Tatakis, D.N. Long-Term Outcomes of Untreated Buccal Gingival Recessions: A Systematic Review and Meta-Analysis. *J. Periodontol.* **2016**, *87*, 796–808. [CrossRef] [PubMed]
16. Joss-Vassalli, I.; Grebenstein, C.; Topouzelis, N.; Sculean, A.; Katsaros, C. Orthodontic Therapy and Gingival Recession: A Systematic Review. *Orthod. Craniofacial. Res.* **2010**, *13*, 127–141. [CrossRef]
17. Bollen, A.M.; Cunha-Cruz, J.; Bakko, D.W.; Huang, G.J.; Hujoel, P.P. The Effects of Orthodontic Therapy on Periodontal Health: A Systematic Review of Controlled Evidence. *J. Am. Dent. Assoc.* **2008**, *139*, 413–422. [CrossRef]
18. Kim, D.M.; Neiva, R. Periodontal Soft Tissue Non–Root Coverage Procedures: A Systematic Review from the AAP Regeneration Workshop. *J. Periodontol.* **2015**, *86*, S56–S72. [CrossRef] [PubMed]
19. Bin Bahar, B.S.K.; Alkhalidy, S.R.; Kaklamanos, E.G.; Athanasiou, A.E. Do Orthodontic Patients Develop More Gingival Recession in Anterior Teeth Compared to Untreated Individuals? A Systematic Review of Controlled Studies. *Int. Orthod.* **2020**, *18*, 1–9. [CrossRef] [PubMed]
20. Jepsen, S.; Caton, J.G.; Albandar, J.M.; Bissada, N.F.; Bouchard, P.; Cortellini, P.; Demirel, K.; de Sanctis, M.; Ercoli, C.; Fan, J.; et al. Periodontal Manifestations of Systemic Diseases and Developmental and Acquired Conditions: Consensus Report of Workgroup 3 of the 2017 World Workshop on the Classification of Periodontal and Peri-Implant Diseases and Conditions. *J. Clin. Periodontol.* **2018**, *45*, S219–S229. [CrossRef] [PubMed]
21. Slutzkey, S.; Levin, L. Gingival Recession in Young Adults: Occurrence, Severity, and Relationship to Past Orthodontic Treatment and Oral Piercing. *Am. J. Orthod. Dentofac. Orthop.* **2008**, *134*, 652–656. [CrossRef]
22. Bechara Andere, N.M.R.; dos Santos, N.C.C.; Araujo, C.F.; Mathias, I.F.; Rossato, A.; de Marco, A.C.; Santamaria, M.; Jardini, M.A.N.; Santamaria, M.P. Evaluation of the Local Effect of Nonsurgical Periodontal Treatment with and without Systemic Antibiotic and Photodynamic Therapy in Generalized Aggressive Periodontitis. A Randomized Clinical Trial. *Photodiagnosis Photodyn Ther.* **2018**, *24*, 115–120. [CrossRef] [PubMed]

23. Aziz, T.; Flores-Mir, C. A Systematic Review of the Association between Appliance-Induced Labial Movement of Mandibular Incisors and Gingival Recession. *Aust. Orthod. J.* **2011**, *27*, 33–39.
24. Ciavarella, D.; Tepedino, M.; Gallo, C.; Montaruli, G.; Zhurakivska, K.; Coppola, L.; Troiano, G.; Chimenti, C.; Laurenziello, M.; Lo Russo, L. Post-Orthodontic Position of Lower Incisors and Gingival Recession: A Retrospective Study. *J. Clin. Exp. Dent.* **2017**, *9*, e1425–e1430. [CrossRef] [PubMed]
25. Yared, K.F.G.; Zenobio, E.G.; Pacheco, W. Periodontal Status of Mandibular Central Incisors after Orthodontic Proclination in Adults. *Am. J. Orthod. Dentofacial. Orthop.* **2006**, *130*, e1–e8. [CrossRef]
26. Pernet, F.; Vento, C.; Pandis, N.; Kiliaridis, S. Long-Term Evaluation of Lower Incisors Gingival Recessions after Orthodontic Treatment. *Eur. J. Orthod.* **2019**, *41*, 559–564. [CrossRef] [PubMed]
27. Renkema, A.M.; Fudalej, P.S.; Renkema, A.; Kiekens, R.; Katsaros, C. Development of Labial Gingival Recessions in Orthodontically Treated Patients. *Am. J. Orthod. Dentofacial. Orthop.* **2013**, *143*, 206–212. [CrossRef]
28. Vasconcelos, G.; Kjellsen, K.; Preus, H.; Vandevska-Radunovic, V.; Hansen, B.F. Prevalence and Severity of Vestibular Recession in Mandibular Incisors after Orthodontic Treatment: A Case-Control Retrospective Study. *Angle Orthod.* **2012**, *82*, 42–47. [CrossRef]
29. Thomson, W.M. Orthodontic Treatment Outcomes in the Long Term: Findings from a Longitudinal Study of New Zealanders. *Angle Orthod.* **2002**, *72*, 449–455.
30. Gebistorf, M.; Mijuskovic, M.; Pandis, N.; Fudalej, P.S.; Katsaros, C. Gingival Recession in Orthodontic Patients 10 to 15 Years Posttreatment: A Retrospective Cohort Study. *Am. J. Orthod. Dentofacial. Orthop.* **2018**, *153*, 645–655. [CrossRef]
31. Morris, J.W.; Campbell, P.M.; Tadlock, L.P.; Boley, J.; Buschang, P.H. Prevalence of Gingival Recession after Orthodontic Tooth Movements. *Am. J. Orthod. Dentofacial. Orthop.* **2017**, *151*, 851–859. [CrossRef]
32. Juloski, J.; Glisic, B.; Vandevska-Radunovic, V. Long-Term Influence of Fixed Lingual Retainers on the Development of Gingival Recession: A Retrospective, Longitudinal Cohort Study. *Angle Orthod.* **2017**, *87*, 658–664. [CrossRef] [PubMed]
33. Sawan, N.M.; Ghoneima, A.; Stewart, K.; Liu, S. Risk Factors Contributing to Gingival Recession among Patients Undergoing Different Orthodontic Treatment Modalities. *Interv. Med. Appl. Sci.* **2018**, *10*, 19–26. [CrossRef] [PubMed]
34. Tepedino, M.; Franchi, L.; Fabbro, O.; Chimenti, C. Post-Orthodontic Lower Incisor Inclination and Gingival Recession—A Systematic Review. *Prog Orthod.* **2018**, *19*, 17. [CrossRef] [PubMed]
35. Grassia, V.; Nucci, L.; Marra, P.M.; Isola, G.; Itro, A.; Perillo, L. Long-Term Outcomes of Nonextraction Treatment in a Patient with Severe Mandibular Crowding. *Case Rep. Dent.* **2020**, *2020*, 1376472. [CrossRef] [PubMed]
36. Kan, J.Y.K.; Morimoto, T.; Rungcharassaeng, K.; Roe, P.; Smith, D.H. Gingival Biotype Assessment in the Esthetic Zone: Visual versus Direct Measurement. *Int. J. Periodontics Restorative Dent.* **2010**, *30*, 237–243.
37. Ainamo, J.; Bay, I. Problems and Proposals for Recording Gingivitis and Plaque. *Int. Dent. J.* **1975**, *25*, 229–235.
38. O'Leary, T.J.; Drake, R.B.; Naylor, J.E. The Plaque Control Record. *J. Periodontol.* **1972**, *43*, 38. [CrossRef]
39. Serino, G.; Wennström, J.L.; Lindhe, J.; Eneroth, L. The Prevalence and Distribution of Gingival Recession in Subjects with a High Standard of Oral Hygiene. *J. Clin. Periodontol.* **1994**, *21*, 57–63. [CrossRef]
40. Pandis, N.; Vlahopoulos, K.; Madianos, P.; Eliades, T. Long-Term Periodontal Status of Patients with Mandibular Lingual Fixed Retention. *Eur. J. Orthod.* **2007**, *29*, 471–476. [CrossRef]
41. Jati, A.S.; Furquim, L.Z.; Consolaro, A. Gingival Recession: Its Causes and Types, and the Importance of Orthodontic Treatment. *Dental Press J. Orthod.* **2016**, *21*, 18–29. [CrossRef]
42. d'Apuzzo, F.; Nucci, L.; Delfino, I.; Portaccio, M.; Minervini, G.; Isola, G.; Serino, I.; Camerlingo, C.; Lepore, M. Application of Vibrational Spectroscopies in the Qualitative Analysis of Gingival Crevicular Fluid and Periodontal Ligament during Orthodontic Tooth Movement. *J Clin. Med.* **2021**, *10*, 1405. [CrossRef] [PubMed]

Review

Dento-Skeletal Class III Treatment with Mixed Anchored Palatal Expander: A Systematic Review

Fabrizia d'Apuzzo [1,†], Ludovica Nucci [1,*,†], Bruno M. Strangio [1], Alessio Danilo Inchingolo [2,*], Gianna Dipalma [2,*], Giuseppe Minervini [1], Letizia Perillo [1,‡] and Vincenzo Grassia [1,‡]

[1] Multidisciplinary Department of Medical-Surgical and Dental Specialties, University of Campania Luigi Vanvitelli, 80138 Naples, Italy; fabrizia.dapuzzo@unicampania.it (F.d.); strangio@protonmail.ch (B.M.S.); giuseppe.minervini@unicampania.it (G.M.); letizia.perillo@unicampania.it (L.P.); grassiavincenzo@libero.it (V.G.)

[2] Interdisciplinary Department of Medicine, University of Bari Aldo Moro, 70124 Bari, Italy

* Correspondence: ludovica.nucci@unicampania.it (L.N.); ad.inchingolo@libero.it (A.D.I.); giannadipalma@tiscali.it (G.D.)

† These authors contributed equally to this work.
‡ These authors contributed equally to this work.

Abstract: Bone-anchored appliances for the treatment of Class III malocclusions have recently been found to reduce the dentoalveolar effects caused by conventional tooth-borne devices while also improving orthopaedic outcomes in growing patients. The goal of this systematic review was to compare the outcomes of skeletal Class III interceptive treatment with dental anchoring devices to those achieved with mixed anchored palatal expanders. The inclusion criteria were as follows: patients who were treated with hybrid anchored palatal expanders and different maxillary advancement appliances. Study quality was estimated using the Newcastle–Ottawa scale. A search on the Pubmed, Scopus, Embase and Cochrane Library databases yielded 350 papers. Following the initial abstract selection, 65 potentially acceptable papers were thoroughly examined, resulting in a final selection of 9 articles. The results in the short-term showed that combined tooth-borne and bone-borne appliances for rapid maxillary expansion might be recommended in protocols of skeletal Class III treatment to obtain more skeletal effects and reduce side effects on the upper teeth.

Keywords: Class III malocclusion; mixed anchored palatal expander; skeletal anchorage; interceptive treatment; systematic review; bone anchorage devices

1. Introduction

The treatment of skeletal Class III malocclusion is sometimes a challenge in orthodontics. The prevalence of this type of malocclusion presents high variability among and within populations ranging from 0% to 26%: the populations from Southeast Asian countries (Chinese and Malaysian) showed the highest prevalence rate of 15.8%, Middle Eastern nations had a mean prevalence rate of 10.2%, European countries had a lower prevalence rate of 4.9% and the Indian population showed the lowest one of 1.2% [1]. The etiology of Class III malocclusion is generally genetic, as has been demonstrated in several studies. [1–3]. A wide range of environmental factors have been suggested as contributing to the onset of Class III malocclusion (enlarged tonsil, difficulty nasal breathing, habit of protruding the mandible) [2–6]. Craniofacial features may be attributed to the incongruity of position and the size of the craniofacial structures at the skull base, maxilla and/or mandible [7–15]. Several tooth-borne anchorage treatments have been proposed to treat Class III dentoskeletal disharmony, including intraoral and extraoral appliances, such as rapid maxillary expansion [16–19] along with the facial mask (RME/FM) and two occlusal acrylic splints associated with Class III elastics and chin-cup (SEC III) [20,21].

Some adverse effects were reported with the use of conventional dental anchorage as RME/FM such as upper incisors proclination and extrusion and mesial tipping of the upper molars, gingival recessions, [3,22–28] fenestrations of the buccal cortex and root resorption of the posterior teeth [29–34]. The SEC III appliances also present some limits, such as uncomfortable dimensions of splints and the impossibility of having expansion in the upper arch. Therefore, a modified SEC III protocol including a maxillary bonded expander has been used with the remaining limit of the mesializing effect of the upper arch [20]. To overcome tooth-borne anchorage treatment limitations, the use of bone anchorage has recently been proposed [10,35–38]. The use of micro-implants allows for the achievement of skeletal anchorage without the need for surgical procedures such as mini-plate placement and removal [39–46]. The goal of this systematic review of the literature is to determine the efficacy of using a mixed anchored palatal expander to treat Class III malocclusions, as well as to see if using a bone-anchorage device induces more maxillary advancement with fewer dental side effects.

2. Materials and Methods

The authors registered this systematic review on PROSPERO, the International Prospective Register of Systematic Reviews (Centre for Reviews and Dissemination, University of York, York, UK). The protocol was under registration at PROSPERO with the number CRD42022207212.

2.1. Search Strategy

The bibliography was rigorously evaluated in accordance with PRISMA 2020 guidelines (Preferred Reporting Items for Systematic Reviews and Meta-Analyses) [17]. Pubmed, Scopus, Embase and Cochrane Library databases were extensively used for research, with no limit in terms of publication date, in September 2021. The keywords include Mesh and non-Mesh terms to limit the field of study. The research strategy was: "skeletal anchorage or bone anchor or miniscrew or mini-implant or bone screw" combined with "skeletal Class III or mandibular prognathism or mandibular hyperplasia or maxillary retrusion or maxillary hypoplasia or mandibular protrusion or Angle Class III" and "interceptive treatment or early treatment or orthopedic treatment or interceptive orthodontic or interceptive or early therapy". These terms were combined in different ways, and further studies cited in the included articles were analyzed.

Title and abstract screening were performed to select articles for full-text retrieval by two reviewers (B.M.S. and L.N.). To find potentially relevant papers, an initial screening of titles and abstracts against the inclusion criteria was undertaken, followed by a review of the complete potentially relevant papers. Duplicate publications were deleted, and studies were chosen for inclusion by both authors separately. The two reviewers had a concordance rate of less than 3%, and any doubts or disputes were resolved following conversation.

2.2. Selection Criteria for the Studies Included in This Review

The inclusion criteria were the following: published articles, articles in press and reviews concerning studies in humans. Randomized clinical trials (RCTs), case–control studies and retrospective and prospective cohort studies were accepted. The exclusion criteria were: case reports, case series, literature reviews, systematic reviews, meta-analyses and editorials and any articles including animal or laboratories studies or patients with syndromes or craniofacial deformities or who had undergone maxillofacial surgery. The eligibility sample criteria were growing patients with skeletal Class III malocclusion who had undergone orthodontic treatment with mixed-anchored palatal expanders.

2.3. Data Collection Process

The variables recorded for each article reviewed were: author, aim, sample size, demographic variables (gender, age), treatment used and the study results. A customized data collection form was created to gather information from the selected studies.

2.4. Types of Outcomes

The primary outcome was the evaluation of skeletal changes after Class III treatment using a mixed anchored palatal expander. The secondary outcome was to compare results obtained using this protocol and others with tooth-borne anchorage.

2.5. Quality Assessment

The Newcastle–Ottawa scale was used by the same researchers to assess the quality of the studies [47]. In case of a disagreement between the two initial researchers, a consensus was reached, and the third researcher was consulted in case of question.

2.6. Risk of Bias Assessment

The evaluation of the risk of bias for the selected studies was carried out independently by B.M.S. and L.N., using the Cochrane Collaboration tool (Figure 1). In case of disagreement, the third author (V.G.) was consulted. A consensus was reached through discussion. Risk of bias rated as "low," "high" or "unclear" included the following: random sequence generation, sample size, allocation concealment, blinding of participants and personnel, blinding of outcome assessment, incomplete outcome data, selective reporting and other biases.

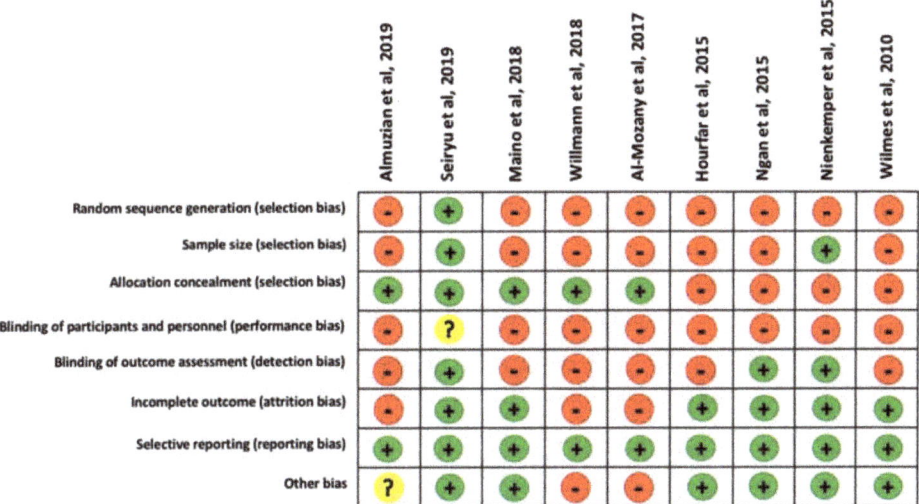

Figure 1. Risk of bias assessed according to Cochrane.

3. Results

3.1. Study Selection and Flow Diagram

The initial search identified a total of 350 articles. After removing 73 duplicates, 277 articles were screened and 226 articles were excluded after reading the title and abstract due to their poor relevance to the research question. The remaining 65 articles were analyzed. Among these, 56 were excluded for these reasons: 13 were case reports, 12 were case series, 1 was an animal study, 9 included adult patients, 5 showed orthognathic surgery, 9 did not use palatal screws and 7 was an in vitro study. At the end, 9 articles were included in the qualitative synthesis (Figure 2).

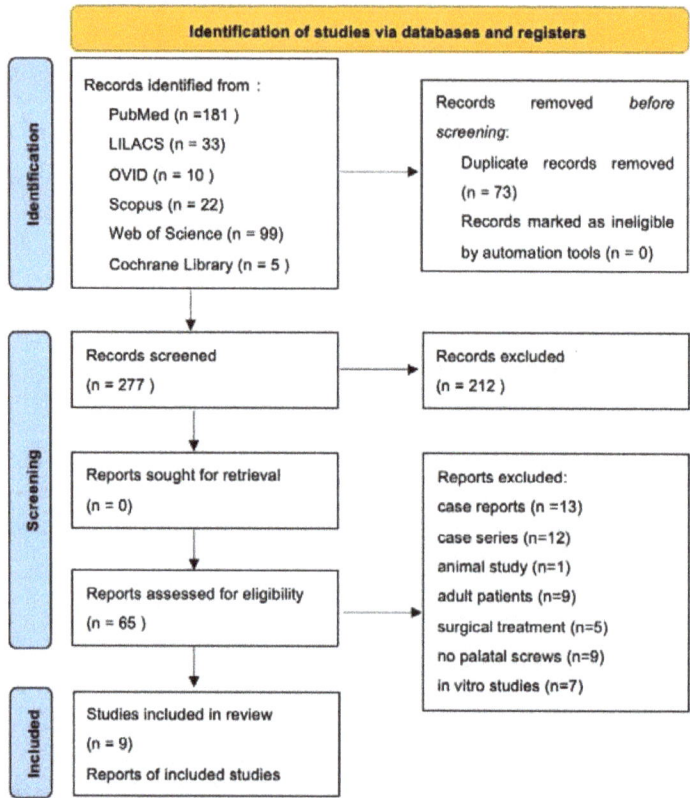

Figure 2. Flow diagram of the selection of the studies (according to PRISMA 2020 flow diagram) [17].

3.2. Study Characteristics

On the Newcastle–Ottawa scale, the 9 studies included in this study had varying levels of quality [25] as shown in Table 1. A total of 5 studies [4,15,29,48–50] presented low to moderate quality, whereas 4 [1,51–53] presented high quality.

Of the 9 studies, one was a randomized clinical trial, 5 were case-control studies and 3 were cohort studies. In 6 studies, a bone-anchored palatal device group was compared with the control one. One of these did not receive any treatment. Another was treated with combined tooth and bone-borne appliances [50]. In two studies, the control groups were treated with tooth-borne appliances and facemasks [52,54], and in the last one, the control group was treated with hybrid Hyrax and mentoplates [53].

The patients' characteristics in the selected studies were: growing phase; skeletal and molar Class III malocclusion; anterior crossbite and/or edge-to-edge occlusion.

3.3. Qualitative Synthesis of the Studies Included

The qualitative analyses of the studies included were performed (Table 2). Al-Mozany et al. [4] and Almuzian et al. [15] selected 14 participants (7 M and 7 F; average age: 12.05 ± 1.09 years) with these features: Cervical Vertebral Maturational (CVM) Stage 2 or 3; retrognathic or hypoplastic maxilla; anterior crossbite and dental Class III molars and canines. The exclusion criteria were: previous orthodontic/orthopedic treatment or congenital abnormalities. All records (T1) were taken in the centric relation before starting the intervention.

Table 1. Studies' quality according to the Newcastle–Ottawa Scale.

Author/Year [Reference]	Selection				Comparability	Exposure		
	Case Definition Adequate	Representativeness of Cases	Selection of Controls	Definition of Controls	Comparability of Cases & Controls	Ascertainment of Exposure	Same Method of Ascertainment	Non-Response Rate
Al-Mozany et al.								
Almuzian et al.		*				*	*	
Wilmes et al.		*				*	*	
Maino et al.		*				*	*	
Nienkemper et al.	*	*	*	*	*	*	*	
Hourfar et al.			*	*	*	*	*	
Seiryu et al.	*		*	*	*	*	*	
Ngan et al.			*	*	*	*	*	
Willmann et al.		*	*	*	*	*	*	

Table 2. Studies involved in the qualitative analysis.

Authors	Aim	C (Cases) Co (Controls)/Mean Age (MA)	Randomized	Control (Yes or Not)	Number and Position of Screw (Appliance Design)	Inclusion Criteria	Methods	Results
Al-Mozany et al./ Almuzian et al.	To evaluate the skeletal and soft tissue effects of the alternate RME and constriction (Alt-Ramec) protocol in conjunction with a miniscrew forgrowing participants with retrognathic maxilla, evaluated by cephalometric analysis (2017) and 3D cone-beam (2019).	Ca (14) MA (12.5 ± 1.9 years)	No	No	MARME with two paramedial palatal TADs and two mandibular TADs, inserted between the canine and the lateral incisor	-Patients at CVM Stage 2 or 3 -Patients with clinically diagnosed retrognathic or hypoplastic maxilla -Anterior crossbite and dental Class III molars and canines	All participants had a MARME appliance that was activated by the Alt-Ramec protocol. Full time Class III elastics, delivering 400 g/side, were then used for maxillary protraction.	-Maxilla protraction (SNA 1.87 ± 1.06°; Vert.T-A 3.29 ± 1.54 mm, $p < 0.001$). -Mandibular retropositioning (SNB-2.03 ± 0.85°; Vert.T-B-3.43 ± 4.47 mm, $p < 0.001$ and $p < 0.05$ respectively) -A significant improvement in the skeletal relationship (ANB 3.95 ± 0.57°, $p < 0.001$). Wits 5.15 ± 1.51 mm, $p < 0.001$) -Increase of Y-axis angle (1.95 ± 1.11°, $p < 0.001$). -The upper incisors precination (+ 2.98 ± 2.71°, $p < 0.01$), coupled with a significant retroclination of the lower incisors (−3.2 ± 3.4°, $p < 0.05$) -A significant improvement in the OVJ (5.62 ± 1.36 mm, $p < 0.001$) and in the Harmony angle (2.76 ± 1.8°, $p < 0.001$)
Wilmes et al.	To assess the clinical applicability and 3D effects of RPE using the hybrid hyrax.	Ca (13) MA (11.2 years)	No	No	Two miniscrews were inserted in the anterior palate next to the midpalatal suture and near the second and third palatal rugae. The miniscrews and two molar bands were used to connect the Hybrid Hyrax device.	-Patients with Class III malocclusion	RPE was performed in 13 patients. In 10 patients with a skeletal Class III occlusion, a facemask was used for maxillary protraction.	-The mean expansion in the first premolar/first primary molar region was 6.3 ± 2.9 mm and 5.0 ± 1.5 mm in the first molar region. -The Wits appraisal changed from −5.2 ± 1.3 mm to −2.5 ± 1.5 mm (mean improvement 2.7 ± 1.3 mm). -The right first molar migrated 0.4 ± 0.6 mm mesially and the left one 0.3 ± 0.2 mm.
Maino et al.	To describe the skeletal and dentoalveolar changes in a group of growing skeletal Class III patients treated with hybrid palatal expander and facemask.	Ca (28) MA (11.4 ± 2.5 years)	No	No	Hybrid palatal expander was connected to two paramedial palatal miniscrews	Growing patient with Class III malocclusion.	28 patients were treated using a rapid maxillary expander with hybrid anchorage according to the ALT-Ramec protocol, followed by 4 months of facemask therapy. Palatal miniscrew placement was accomplished via digital planning and the construction of a high-precision individualized surgical guide.	-Point A advanced by a mean of 3.4 mm with respect to the reference plane Vert-T. -The mandibular plane rotated clockwise, improving the ANB (+3.41°) and the Wits appraisal (+4.92 mm). -The maxillary first molar had slight extrusion (0.42 mm) and mesialization (0.87 mm).

41

Table 2. Cont.

Authors	Aim	C (Cases) Co (Controls)/Mean Age (MA)	Randomized	Control (Yes or Not)	Number and Position of Screw (Appliance Design)	Inclusion Criteria	Methods	Results
Nienkemper et al.	To value the efficacy of hybrid hyrax and facemask (FM) combination in growing Class III patients.	Ca (16) MA (9.5 ± 1.6 years) Co (16) MA (9.4 ± 1.1 years)	No	Yes	On both sides of the midpalatal suture, two micro implants were placed in the anterior palate. The miniscrews and two molar bands were used to connect the Hybrid hyrax device. To apply the protraction, two rigid sectional wires were welded to the buccal side of the molar bands.	Class III malocclusion in the mixed dentition characterized by a Wits index of −2 mm or less (mean, −5.6 ± 2.2 mm) -Anterior crossbite or incisor edge-to-edge relationship -Class III molar relationship -CVM (CS1-3)	16 growing Class III patients were treated with a RPE with a hybrid hyrax. A facemask was used to perform a maxillary protraction. A control group of 16 untreated Class III participants was compared to the treatment group.	-SNA and Point A to nasion perpendicular showed significant increments of 2.4° and 2.4 mm, respectively -A significant reduction in the length and sagittal position of the mandible (CoGn −2.3 mm and SNB −1.7°) -The Wits index augmented by 4.5 mm and the ANB improved by 4.1° -Co-Go-Me angle decrease significantly (2.0°). No significant increase of FM∆ (0.5°) -OVJ and molar relationship improved significantly (3.2 mm and −3.1 mm, respectively) -No significant differences could be found in OVB or inclination of the maxillary and mandibular incisors.
Hourfar et al.	To compare cephalometric changes after treatment with two types of fast maxillary expansion appliances: a tooth-borne appliance and a tooth-and-bone-borne appliance.	Ca (50); MA (13.04 ± 4.82 years) Co (50) MA (13.04 ± 4.82 years)	No	Yes	Two miniscrews were placed in the anterior palate at paramedian locations. These miniscrews held the anterior side of a hybrid hyrax, while the posterior side was attached to the molar bands on the front molars.	-Patients treated with strictly tooth-borne or patients treated with combined tooth- and bone-borne appliances -Skeletal Class I (0° < ANB ≤ 4°) or Class III (ANB ≤ 0°) -Bilateral posterior crossbite	Cephalometry was used to examine the pre- and post-treatment lateral cephalograms of 100 patients. 50 of the patients were treated with exclusively tooth-borne appliances, whereas the other 50 were treated with a combination of tooth-and-bone-borne appliances. Additional sub-groups were constructed based on pre-treatment cephalometric data for skeletal Class I or Class III to detect any implications for clinical therapy.	-Pronounced anterior shift of the maxilla (SNA increase by 2°) -Caudal shift of the maxilla -Upper jaw inclination remained almost the same. -Increases in the vertical parameters ML/NSL (1.46°) and Björk sum (1.46).
Seirya et al.	To investigate difference in treatment outcomes of milder skeletal Class III malocclusion between FM and FM + MS in growing patients	Ca (20) MA (10.05 ± 1.8 years) Co (19) MA (11 ± 1.3 years)	Yes	Yes	In the FM + MS group, one miniscrew was inserted in the anterior region of the palate. A lingual arch with soldered hooks was attached to the miniscrew.	-Skeletal class III (ANB ≤ 2.5°) -OVJ ≥ 0 -CVMS II–IV -No congenital or systemic disease -No skeletal asymmetry -No missing teeth -No temporomandibular joint disorder	A lingual arch with hooks was fixed to the maxillary arch in both groups and a protrusive force of 500 g was applied form the FM to the hooks, 12 hours per day.	-No MS mobility or loss during treatment -Cephalometric analysis showed a significant increase in SNA (1.1°), SN-ANS (1.3°), and ANB (0.8°) in the FM + MS group -Proclination of maxillary incisors significantly greater in the FM group (4.6°)
Ngan et al.	The goal of this study was to examine the skeletal and dentoalveolar alterations in patients treated with tooth-borne Hyrax +FM versus hybrid Hyrax + FM.	Ca (20) MA (9.8 ± 1.6 years) Co (20) MA (9.6 ± 1.2 years)	No	Yes	In the hybrid Hyrax group two Benefit micro-implants were placed in the third palatal rugae.	-Class III malocclusion: -Anterior crossbite or edge-to-edge incisal relationship -Wits ≤ −3/ANB ≤ −2°	A total of 20 patients were treated with tooth-borne Hyrax + FM, while 20 patients were treated with bone-borne Hyrax +FM in a row. The screw was activated twice daily by the patients in both groups for one week, and then two weeks when a constricted maxillary was evident. Maxillary protraction was performed with 380 g per side elastics for 12-14 hours per day.	-Sagittal relationship improved in both groups; tooth-borne (Wits 2.19, ANB 2.58°) and bone-borne (Wits 2.31 mm, ANB 2.17°). -Greater downward movement of the maxilla in tooth-borne (OLp-A pt. 1.2 mm) compared to bone-borne (−0.4 mm, p < 0.05) -Forward and backward movement of the mandible in both groups (OLp-A pt, 0.7 mm/2.2 mm) -Mandibular plane angle was found to open more in tooth-borne (SNL-ML 2.76°) compared to bone-borne (−0.25°, p < 0.05) -Greater change in OVJ in the tooth-borne group (5.5 mm) compared to the bone-anchored group (3.4 mm, p < 0.001) -Greater forward movement of maxillary incisors in the tooth-borne group (OLp-Is 2.12 vs. 0.87, p < 0.05) and greater differential maxillary/mandibular molars movement
Willmann et al.	To compare skeletal and dental effects of hybrid Hyrax + FM and hybrid Hyrax + Mentoplate (MP)	Ca (17) MA (8.74 ± 1.20 years) Co (17) MA (9.43 ± 0.95 years)	No	Yes	Hybrid Hyrax devices were fitted on two paramedian mini-implants in the anterior palate. Mentoplate was inserted subapical to the lower incisors.	-Wits ≤ −2.0 mm -From 7 to 12 years -Anterior crossbite or incisor edge-to-edge relationship -Molar class III relationship	34 patients were treated with Hybrid Hyrax. In 17, maxillary protraction was performed with FM, while the other 17 were treated in combination with MP. The expander screw was activated 4 times/day; the FM group wore 400 g elastics on each side 14-16 h per day while the MP full-time.	-Significant forward movement of A-point (FM GROUP: SNA + 2.23° ± 1.30° — p 0.000°; ME: 2.23° ± 1.43° — p 0.000°); -B-Point showed a larger sagittal change in the FM Group (SNB 1.51 ± 1.1° — p 0.000°) compared to the ME group (SNB- 0.30 ± 0.9° — p 0.070); -FM group showed a significant increase in the ML-NL + 1.86 ± 1.65° (p 0.000°) and NSL-ML + 1.17 ± 1.48 (p 0.006°); -Upper incisor inclination as well as the distance of the first upper Molar in relation to A-point did not change significantly in both groups.

Maino et al. [49] selected 28 patients (15 males and 13 females; mean age: 11.4 ± 2.5 years). The inclusion criteria were: growing phase; Class III malocclusion (evaluating Wits index). The exclusion criteria were craniofacial syndromes and previous orthopedic or orthodontic treatment. Wilmes et al. [29] selected 13 patients (7 females and 6 males; mean age: 11.2 years), but they did not report the inclusion and exclusion criteria. Nienkemper et al. [51] selected a treatment group of 16 patients and a control group of 16 untreated patients. At the start (T1), all patients showed mixed dentition, with a Wits index of –2 mm or less (mean, −5.6 ± 2.2 mm), anterior crossbite or incisor edge-to-edge relationship and a Class III molar relationship. According to the Cervical Vertebral Maturation method, all patients were in the prepubertal stage of skeletal maturity (CS1-3). Hourfar et al. [50] selected 100 patients (59 females and 41 males; mean age: 13.04 ± 4.82 years) with transverse deficits of the maxilla; all had been treated by RME without surgical support in the context of orthodontic treatment indications. A total of 2 groups of 50 patients were formed, including a conventional group of 29 females/21 males treated with strictly tooth-borne appliances and a hybrid group of 30 females/20 males treated with appliances anchored in both the teeth and jawbone. The patients were further divided into the skeletal Class I ($0° < ANB \leq 4°$) or Class III ($ANB \leq 0°$) subgroup based on their pretreatment cephalometric findings. The other inclusion criteria were Caucasian descent and bilateral posterior crossbite. The exclusion criteria were: previous orthodontic treatment, the extraction of permanent teeth, planned extractions, congenital agenesis of permanent teeth, craniofacial anomalies or trauma, systemic disease, trauma of frontal teeth with or without tooth loss, or maxillary protraction (facemask). Seiryu et al. [55] selected 39 patients, 20 treated only with facemasks (FM group) and 19 treated with facemasks and miniscrews (FM + MS group). Ngan et al. [54] selected 40 Class III patients, 20 of whom received the tooth-borne maxillary RPE and protraction device and 20 of whom received a bone-anchored maxillary RPE and protraction appliances. Willmann et al. [53] selected 34 patients for hybrid hyrax appliance treatment, 17 for the facemask (mean age 8.74 ± 1.20) and the other 17 for mentoplate (mean age 9.43 ± 0.95) for maxillary advancement.

3.4. Skeletal Anchorage

Various methods have been used, which excluded any skeletal anchorage: Maino et al. [49] treated patients using a rapid palatal expander (RPE) with hybrid anchorage. Two paramedial palatal miniscrews were inserted; the RPE's anterior metal arms were welded to two metal abutments that fit over the miniscrews' heads. Al-Mozany et al. [4] and Almuzian et al. [15] inserted two paramedial palatal miniscrews and two mandibular miniscrews between the canine and lateral incisors. The Hybrid MARME was cemented with a glass ionomer cement on day 28 of the miniscrew insertion. The MLA (modified lingual arch) was built and cemented. The lingual cleats that protruded from the MLA were attached with composite resin to the lingual surfaces of the anterior teeth. Wilmes et al. [29] applied two mini-implants in the anterior palate next to the midpalatal suture and near the second and third palatal rugae. Then, 7 to 10 days after placing the mini-implants, the hybrid hyrax appliance was inserted and connected to the miniscrews and the first permanent molars. Nienkemper et al. [51] placed two mini-implants on opposite sides of the midpalatal suture in the anterior part. A split palatal screw, two orthodontic bands attached to the first molars and two abutments screwed to mini-implants made up the hybrid hyrax appliance. Rigid stainless-steel wire with a diameter of 1.5 mm was used to connect these components. Rigid sectional wires were soldered to the buccal side of the molar bands to apply orthopedic protraction forces. Hourfar et al. [50] used two miniscrews in the anterior palate at paramedian locations. These miniscrews supported the anterior side of a hybrid hyrax, while the posterior side was connected to the orthodontic bands on the first molars, with RME force applied via a centrally located expansion screw. Seiryu et al. [55] inserted a miniscrew in the anterior region of the palate. Ngan et al. [54] placed two mini-implants in the area of the third palatal rugae. Willman et al. [53] placed two paramedian screws in the anterior palate to fit a Hybrid-Hyrax, while in patients treated with mentoplates, the device was inserted in the subapical region of the lower incisors.

3.5. Expansion Activation Protocol

Maino et al. [49] used a RME with hybrid anchorage according to the Alt-Ramec protocol (alternation of expansion and compression of the maxillary complex). Al-Mozany et al. [4] and Almuzian et al. [15] also used the Alt-Ramec protocol. Wilmes et al. [29] activated the sagittal split screw twice a day by a 90° turn immediately after insertion of the hybrid hyrax. This resulted in a daily activation of 0.8 mm. RPE was continued until a 30% overcorrection was achieved. The split screw was activated by 90° turns 4 times/day by Nienkemper et al. [51], resulting in an expansion of 0.8 mm/day. The activation was continued until a 30% transverse overcorrection was obtained. Hourfar et al. [50] activated the expansion screw of the RME appliance 3 times/day for a change of 0.2 mm per activation. Seiryu et al. [55] used a screw to support a lingual arch, and no expansion device was used. Ngan et al. [54] instructed patients to activate the jackscrew twice daily for one week, whereas patients with constricted maxilla activated for two weeks. Willman et al. [53] performed the RME activating the screw four times a day.

3.6. Class III Biomechanics

Maino et al. [49]: maxillary protraction was achieved via facemask, which was to be worn 14 h per day for 4 months. The protraction elastics (400 g per side) were attached near the maxillary canines, with a downward and forward pull of 30° from the occlusal plane. Al-Mozany et al. [4], Almuzian et al. [15]: prescription was written for two full-time heavy intra-oral elastics per side, totaling 400 g per side One of these elastics ran in the long-closing Class III configuration, from the posterior ball clasps on the hybrid MARPE to the "S" hook. The other ran from the anterior hook on the hybrid MARPE to the MLA in a short-closing Class III configuration. In Wilmes et al. [26] a facemask was prescribed for approximately 6 months to simultaneously protract the maxilla. The applied elastics (142 g) were anterocaudally angulated. Facemasks were used by Nienkemper et al. [51] to achieve maxillary protraction. The elastics were applied with an inclination in both directions (downward and forward) of 20–30° from the occlusal plane. The elastics delivered 400 g of force per side, which was controlled by a force gauge. The patients were told to wear the facemask for 16 h/day. Hourfar et al. [50] used only a RPE, with no sagittal force directed on the maxilla. Seiryu et al. [55] applied a protractive force of 250 g per side from the facemask to the hooks using elastics. The FM has been worn for 12 h per day with a direction of traction force < 3° from the occlusal plane. Ngan et al. [54] attached heavy elastics to generate the maxillary advancement, which delivered 380 g per side. The prescription was FM for 12–14 h a day. Willman et al. [53] instructed the facemask patients to wear 400 g elastics per side for 14–16 h per day, adjusting the force vector to have an inclination of 20–30° to the occlusal plane.

3.7. Dentoalveolar Effects

Al-Mozany et al. [4] and Almuzian et al. [15] found a significant proclination of the maxillary incisors (UI-SN +2.98 ± 2.71°, $p < 0.01$) and a retroclination of the mandibular incisors (LI-MP −3.2 ± 3.4°, $p < 0.05$). Maino et al. [49] documented that the maxillary molar had slight extrusion (U6 vert PP 0.42 mm) and mesialization (U6 mesialization 0.87 mm). The average forward displacement of the incisors was 3.62 mm (Pr-VertT), and their retroclination was 2.26° with respect to the palatal plane (U1-PP), according to Maino et al. [49]. Wilmes et al. [29] documented only a mesial migration of the maxillary incisors. The right first molar migrated 0.4 ± 0.6 mm mesially and the left one 0.3 ± 0.2 mm. In addition, Al-Mozany et al. and Almuzian et al. [4,15] recorded a significant improvement in the overjet: 5.63 ± 1.36 mm ($p < 0.001$). Both the manuscripts of Maino and Wilmes [29,49] did not report the values of OVJ and OVB. Nienkemper et al. [51] recorded a significant improvement in the OVJ and molar relationship (3.2 mm and −3.1 mm, respectively) in the treatment group, but no significant differences between the treatment group and control group (untreated Class III subjects) could be found in OVB (−0.2 mm) or inclination of the maxillary (U1-PP: −0.5°) and mandibular incisors (L1-MP: −1.7°). Hourfar et al. [50] did not analyze the dentoalveolar effects of the hybrid hyrax but only the skeletal effects by pre- and post-treatment lateral cephalograms of the patients. Seiryu et al. [55] referred a major proclination of the maxillary incisors in the FM group in comparison to the FM + MS group (FM group: 4.6 ± 4.5°; FM + MS group: −0.4 ± 4.2°; $p < 0.01$), due to the greater improvement of the skeletal relationship in patients treated with palatal anchorage. Ngan et al. [54] found significant and greater change in OVJ in the tooth-borne group (5.5) compared to the bone-anchored group (3.4 mm, $p < 0.001$). This is due to the tooth-borne group having more forward migration of the maxillary incisors (OLp-Is 2.12 vs. 0.87 mm, $p < 0.05$). Maxillary incisors presented a significantly greater downward movement and palatal inclination in the bone-anchored group (Is-NL 1.34 mm, Is-SNL −4.42°) compared to the tooth-borne group (−0.55 mm, −0.19°, $p < 0.05$). Furthermore, the tooth-borne protraction facemask group had a significant and bigger change in molar relationship (2.7 mm) than the bone-anchored group (1.1 mm, $p < 0.05$), which was due to a greater differential movement of maxillary and mandibular molars in the tooth-borne group. Willman et al. [53] found no statistically significant difference in upper incisor proclination, space loss for the canines and mesial migration of the molars between the study groups. The majority of the overjet correction (FM group 3.51 mm, ME group 3.06 mm) was attributable to skeletal effects rather than dentoalveolar compensation.

3.8. Skeletal Effects

In sagittal dimension, Al-Mozany et al., Almuzian et al. and Dekel et al. [4,15,56] showed maxillary protraction (SNA 1.87 ± 1.06°; Vert.T-A 3.29 ± 1.54 mm $p < 0.001$), whereas the mandibular base significantly retropositioned (SNB −2.03° ± 0.85°; Vert.T-B −3.43 ± 4.47 mm, $p < 0.001$ and $p < 0.05$, respectively), resulting in a better skeletal relationship (ANB 3.95° ± 0.57°, $p < 0.001$; Wits 5.15 ± 1.51 mm, $p < 0.001$). Maino et al. [49] also showed a maxillary advancement (SNA +2.50°; Vert.T-A +3.4 mm), while the mandibular base redirected posteriorly (SNB −0.92°; Vert.T-B −0.26 mm). The mandibular plane rotated clockwise, improving the ANB (+ 3.41°) and the Wits index (+ 4.92 mm). Wilmes et al. [29] did not consider these parameters but specified only an improvement of Wits appraisal (2.7 ± 1.3 mm) and an expansion in the first premolar/first primary molar region and in the first molar region (+ 6.3 ± 2.9 mm and +5.0 ±1.5 mm, respectively). Nienkemper et al. [51] recorded an increase of 2.4° and 2.4 mm SNA and A point to Nasion perpendicular, respectively. Moreover, a significant reduction in CoGn (−2.3 mm) and SNB (−1.7°) was recorded. The Wits index increased by 4.5 mm, and the ANB angle improved by 4.1°. Hourfar et al. [50] recorded an SNA increase of 2°, and the maxilla underwent statistically significant amounts of caudal movement (S-Spa: +3.20; S-Spp: +1.21; N-Spa: +1.84; N-Spp: +2.89), whereas the maxillary inclination had not changed (NL/NSL: −0.06°). Furthermore, a mean mandibular post-rotation was assessed (ML/NSL: +1.46).

For the vertical measurements, Maino et al. [49] recorded that the facial angle (SN-GoGn) increased by 1.64° during treatment and the SN-PP angle was reduced by 1.11°. Al-Mozany et al. and Almuzian et al. [4,15] indicated Y-axis and lower third (ANS-Me) significant increases (1.95 ± 1.22° and 3.19 ± 2.2 mm, respectively), indicating a post-rotation of the mandible. The middle facial height (N-ANS) (0.32 ± 1.53 mm) showed no significant increase. Nienkemper et al. [51] reported that vertical growth was contained as indicated by a slight increase in the FMA angle (0.5°) and a little reduction in the Co-Go-Me angle (2.0°). The other skeletal vertical values showed no significant differences. Hourfar et al. [50] revealed increases in the vertical parameters ML/NSL (+1.46) and Björk sum (+1.46). Seiryu et al. [55] reported that both FM and FM + MS patients showed a significant increase in maxillary forward growth without mandibular forward growth. During the active treatment, SNA (FM + MS group: 2.28 ± 1.38; FM group: 1.18 ± 1.08; $p < 0.01$), SN-ANS (FM + MS group: 2.58 ± 1.78; FM group:1.28 ± 1.38; $p < 0.05$) and ANB (FM + MS group: 2.08 ± 1.38; FM group: 1.28 ± 1.28; $p < 0.05$) change was significantly greater in the FM + MS group than in the FM group.

Ngan et al. [54] found similar maxillary advancement (OLp-A pt., 0.7 mm) and mandible retropositioning (OLp-Pg, 2.2 mm) in both groups. Both the tooth-borne (Wits 2.19 mm, ANB 2.58°) and the bone-anchored (Wits 2.31 mm, ANB 2.17°) groups improved their anteroposterior jaw relationship. Other than that, the tooth-borne (OLparallel–A pt. 1.2 mm) protraction facemask group had a substantially larger downward displacement of the maxilla than the bone-anchored protraction facemask group (−0.4 mm, $p < 0.005$). The tooth-borne group had a considerably higher mandibular plane angle (SNL–ML 2.76°) than the bone-anchored protraction face-mask group (−0.25°, 0.23°, $p < 0.05$). Willman et al. [53] reported a significant improvement in the maxillary position in both groups. Similar changes in the SNA-Angle (SNA + 2.23°) and WITS-appraisal (FM Group 4.81 mm, ME 4.14 mm) during a comparable treatment period were found, while an SNB angle decrease difference was found in the study groups. In the FM-group, the skeletal effect on the mandible is more vertical, as evidenced by a posterior rotation of the mandible and a significant opening of the interbase angle (ML-NL). In the ME-group, however, the B-point remained stable, while the gonial angle decreased significantly, possibly due to changes in condylar and ramus growth (Table 3).

Table 3. Dentoskeletal cephalometric results.

Authors	SNA	SNB	ANB	OVB	OVJ	WITS	SN^GoMe or Equivalents	Upper Incisor Position	Lower Incisor Position
Al-Mozany et al./ Almuzian et al.	1.87 ± 1.06°	2.02 ± 0.85°	3.95 ± 0.57°	1.21 ± 1.89 mm	5.63 ± 1.36 mm	5.16 ± 1.5 mm	Y-axis: 1.95° ± 1.11°	UI-PP:2.98 ± 2.71°	LI-MP:3.2 ± 3.4°
Wilmes et al.	na	na	na	na	na	2.7 ± 1.3 mm	na	na	na
Maino et al.	+2.50°	−0.92°	+3.41°	na	na	+4.92 mm	SN-GoGn: +1.64°	U1-PP: −2.26° Pr-VertT: +3.62 mm	na
Nienkemper et al.	2.4°	−1.7°	4.1°	−0.2 mm	3.2 mm	4.5 mm	Co-Go-Me: −2.0°	U1-PP: −0.5°	L1-MP: −1.7°
Hourfar et al.	2.17°	−0.97°	+2.77°	na	na	na	ML./NSL: 1.46°	na	na
Seiryu et al.	+2.2 ± 1.3°	+0.1 ± 1.3	+2.0 ± 1.3	na	na	na	MP-SN: −0.1 ± 1.3	UI-SN: −0.4 ± 4.2	na
Ngan et al.	1.59°	−0.8°	+2.4°	−0.14 mm	+3.46 mm	+2.58 mm	SNL-ML: +0.24°	Is-SNL: −2.03	li-ML: −1.67
Willmann et al.	FM: 2.23 ± 1.30 MP: 2.23 ± 1.43	FM: −1.51 ± 1.13 MP: −0.30 ± 0.98	FM: 3.75 ± 1.45 MP: 2.54 ± 0.99	na	na	FM: 4.81 ± 1.38 MP: 4.14 ± 1.25	ML-NSL: FM: 1.17 ± 1.48 MP: −0.55 ± 1.09	U1-PP°: FM: −1.15 ± 6.45 MP: 0.57 ± 5.49	L1-ML°: FM: −3.84 ± 6.13 MP: 0.56 ± 3.83

3.9. Soft Tissue Analysis

In Al-Mozany and Almuzian's [15,57] study, cephalometric analysis of soft tissues revealed a significant increase in the H angle, at 2.76° ± 1.8° ($p < 0.001$). None of the remaining authors [26,46–51] reported soft tissue effects.

3.10. Quality Assessment

Al-Mozany et al., Almuzian et al. and Maino et al. [15,49,57] did not have a control group, and the patients were not randomized. Wilmes et al. [29] was a randomized study with a control group of 10 subjects. Nienkemper et al. [51] was a controlled clinical study with a control group of 16 subjects. It was not a randomized study. Hourfar et al. [50] was a retrospective cephalometric study with a control group of 50 subjects. It was not a randomized study. Al-Mozany et al. and Almuzian et al. [15,57] specified that no sample size calculation was undertaken. Maino et al., Wilmes et al. and Hourfar et al. [29,49,50] did not report a power analysis. Nienkemper et al. [58] specified that prior pilot research was used to calculate the sample size calculation. Based on a significant increase in SNA of 2.0° with a σ of 1.9°, an α level of 0.05 and a power of 0.80, the required sample size was found to be 16 patients in the treatment and control groups, respectively. Al-Mozany et al. and Almuzian et al. [15,57], in the section of the statistical analysis, reported that a paired-sample t-test ($p < 0.05$) was used to compare each variable from T1 to T2, and an error measurement (Dahlberg's formula) study was conducted to evaluate the intra-examiner reliability, while, Maino et al. [49] used the Student t-test to check whether the pretreatment and post-treatment variations were significant ($p < 0.05$). Wilmes et al. [29] did not report a statistical analysis. According to Nienkemper et al., the data did not demonstrate normal distribution in an exploratory analysis using the Shapiro–Wilk test [58]. As a result, nonparametric statistics were applied. The Mann-Whitney U-test was used to look for significant differences between the cephalometric variables in the treatment and control groups at T1 (comparison of beginning forms) and during the T1-T2 interval. Hourfar et al. [50] performed paired t-tests for the intragroup and analysis of variance (ANOVA) for the intergroup comparisons. At $p < 0.05$, the results were considered statistically significant.

The research study design used by Seiryu [55] was a single-center, prospective randomized clinical trial. The sample size was calculated using data from a previous study that compared the treatment effects of a combination of bone-anchored maxillary protraction (BAMP) and facemask with a rapid maxillary expander (RME/FM) for maxillary advancement. With a test power of 80%, a significance level of 5% and an effect size of 0.98, the authors reported that treatment with facemask therapy and miniscrews resulted in 1.5 times increase in maxillary forward growth. For each group, a sample size of 18 patients was recommended. A computer-generated 1:1 randomization was carried out by someone who was not involved in the study. To check for normal distribution, all values were subjected to the Shapiro–Wilk test. Welch's t-test was used to assess the significance of differences in all values that showed normal distribution (age, treatment period, cephalometric variables), while the Mann-Whitney U-tests were used to assess those that did not. * $p < 0.05$, ** $p < 0.01$ were used to indicate statistical significance.

Ngan et al. [54] used a two-tailed t-test with a confidence level of 95% to compare the starting forms of the control and experimental samples, as well as the skeletal and dental alterations between the groups at the two time periods. The reliability of cephalometric readings was determined using the intraclass correlation coefficient of reliability (R). All cephalometric variables had correlations ranging from 0.96 to 0.99, with the majority exceeding 0.98 (R value greater than 0.90 indicating high reliability). Willman et al. [53] used the Shapiro–Wilk test to examine the normal distribution of the measurements. Student's t-test for dependent samples or the Wilcoxon test were used to find intra-group differences. The Mann–Whitney U test or the t-test for independent samples were used to test the differences between the groups. The 95% confidence of interval was chosen.

4. Discussion

The purpose of this systematic review of the literature was to determine the effectiveness of treating Class III malocclusions using a mixed anchored palatal expander [56]. Due to a scarcity of studies on this issue, only nine publications, largely case series, were chosen for the following work (characterized by a high research specificity and innovative protocol aspect).

All of the studies that were analyzed include in their protocol an RME appliance applied on a mini-screw anteriorly in the palate to obtain skeletal anchorage. Since the first molars are also included in the device design, it can be denominated as a bone- and tooth-borne appliance (hybrid hyrax). Al-Mozany et al., Almuzian et al. and Maino et al. [4,15,49] employed the Alt-Ramec protocol, which resulted in a more significant disarticulation of the two parts of the maxilla than the other methods of maxillary expansion examined in this research.

Because the ability of sutures to respond to therapy decreases with age, it has been suggested that starting maxillary traction with a facemask during the early mixed dentition period (around 8 years old) will provide the most skeletal benefit [47]. Skeletal anchorage, on the other hand, is treated at a later age, around 10 years old, when the characteristics of the bone allow for easier placement and stability [57]. When compared to pure bone-borne RPE devices such as distractors, the hybrid hyrax is surgically minimally invasive, and this is also important to avoid any periodontal inflammation [58–61]. The use of first molars and mini-screws as, respectively, anterior and posterior anchoring units has various advantages. In fact, according to Wilmes et al. [29], the hybrid hyrax can be employed even in individuals who have decreased anterior dental anchoring owing to missing primary molars, primary molars with resorbed roots or underdeveloped premolar roots. Moreover, the anterior teeth are excluded in the appliance, and regular orthodontic treatment can, therefore, be started early. Furthermore, in all tests, the miniscrews were implanted at paramedian sites in the anterior palate. This configuration is particularly beneficial for bone availability and safe isolation from vascular and nerve connections. The optimal size and direction of miniscrew insertions are identified on a cone-bean computed tomography (CBCT) scan and a 3-dimensional surgical guide to provide safe and reliable palatal miniscrew insertion [49].

Another significant benefit is that the combination of the hybrid hyrax with a maxillary protraction facemask is helpful to minimize dental adverse effects, such as teeth mesial migration. Al-Mozany et al. and Almuzian et al. [4,15] specify that the teeth were partially implicated in the maxillary protraction utilizing hybrid hyrax for the transfer of forces to the underlying skeletal systems. The frequent unfavorable consequences of tooth-anchorage devices, such as buccal proclination of the upper incisors and lingual inclination of the lowers, are eliminated with this procedure. As a result, the therapy had both skeletal and dentoalveolar effects (maxilla protraction and mandible posterior displacement).

Furthermore, the upper incisors displayed a forward displacement of 3.62 mm (Pr-VertT) and a retroclination of 2.26 degrees in reference to the palatal plane (U1-PP), according to Maino et al. [49]. It is likely that the retroclination found in many patients treated with a bone-anchored facemask or hybrid tooth-skeletal anchoring is due to the treatment's skeletal benefits and the resultant diminution of the no-longer-required dentoalveolar compensation. However, despite the anchorage provided by the two mini-screws, Maino et al. [49] assessed the forward movement of the maxillary molars (although by less than 1 mm in all cases). The hybrid hyrax, according to Wilmes et al. [29], minimized excessive forward movement of the upper molars produced by facemask protraction (1.6 migrated 0.4 ± 0.6 mm mesially and 2.6 0.3 ± 0.2 mm). Nienkemper validated these findings, recording a modest molar mesial migration (approximately 0.4 mm) [51].

In the Nienkemper et al. [55], Al-Mozany et al. and Almuzian et al. [15,51] studies, the OVJ was improved. Nienkemper et al. confirmed that the OVB had not improved significantly, although Al-Mozany et al. claimed an improvement in the results section, but this did not match the data in the final table. Because Maino et al., Wilmes et al. and Hourfar et al. [29,49,50] did not show the OVB and OVJ values, it is difficult to know for sure how the OVB and the OVJ changed after therapy with a hybrid palatal expander. The rise in the angle SNA and the Wits assessment revealed a considerable skeletal improvement at the maxillary in the sagittal plane. These values are higher than those obtained with dental anchorage, indicating that skeletal anchorage is superior to dental anchorage because the exerted force was supported by a skeletal component as well as by teeth.

Furthermore, all studies indicated a posterior mandibular rotation using their approach (except Wilmes et al. [29], who did not evaluate the location of the jaw).

These combined, which include maxillary advancement, maxillary caudal movement and a posteriorly shifted mandibular base, reflect a pattern of three-dimensional geometric change that, according to Hourfar et al. [50], has the potential to facilitate the treatment of skeletal Class III patients, but the mandibular clockwise rotation is also a compensation for the treatment of Class III malocclusions [50]. Finally, patients who had mixed anchorage with miniscrews had higher maxillary protraction, which reduced unfavorable dental consequences. The fact that the orthopedic force acts directly on the surrounding sutures, increases the skeletal impact and eliminates dental compensation is one probable explanation [52]. However, these results will need to be verified with more randomized clinical trials and long-term follow-up. According to Seiryu et al. [55], the FM + MS group's proclination of the maxillary anterior teeth at T1 was reduced at T2 by improving the maxilla–mandibular relationship. When compared to orthopedic force alone, the use of miniscrews [52] had fewer negative side effects on the maxillary teeth. As a result, whereas mandibular growth was driven forward and lower, neither clockwise rotation nor posterior displacement of the mandible occurred, showing that face-mask treatment with a miniscrew caused less posterior displacement than miniplates and elastics [55].

Ngan et al. [54] and Willman et al. [53] found that both the tooth-borne and bone-borne groups had identical maxillary protraction; however, Seiryu et al. [55] found that the maxillary protraction in the miniscrew group was bigger by twofold. This discrepancy could be due to the appliance utilized, the treatment length or the age at which the treatment began.

The tooth-born protraction facemask group had more forward movement of the maxillary than the bone-anchored protraction facemask group, resulting in a bigger rise in the OVJ, according to Ngan et al. [54]. Despite the anchorage, the maxillary molars migrated forward by an average of 0.6 mm in the bone-anchored groups; this was most likely due to wire bending rather than mini-implant movement. By combining retroposition of the mandible with advancement of the maxilla, both the tooth-borne and bone-anchored groups (SNB −2.2° and −1.3°, respectively) enhanced Wits evaluation and ANB changes. The miniscrews, on the other hand, help to limit the downward movement of the maxilla and, as a result, the clock-wise rotation of the mandible in the bone-anchored group. Furthermore, the bone-anchored group had more downward movement of the maxillary incisors than the tooth-borne group, contributing to the bone-anchored group's preservation of the OVB.

In Willman et al. [53] study positive skeletal modifications rather than dentoalveolar compensation were shown to be responsible for the majority of the overjet correction (FM group 3.51 mm, ME group 3.06 mm). While the skeletal effects on the maxilla were similar in both groups, the SNB angle was significantly reduced. In the FM group, the interbase angle was observed to be more opened, caused by a posterior rotation of the mandible, which might be due to the chincup of the FM. The B point remains constant in the MP-group, while the gonial angle declines considerably, owing to condylar development redirection [53].

5. Conclusions

According to the nine studies included in this systematic review, combining tooth-borne and bone-borne appliances for rapid maxillary extension may be advised in treatment protocols for skeletal Class III patients to obtain more skeletal results while lowering maxillary dentition side effects.

Author Contributions: Conceptualization, V.G. and L.P.; methodology, F.d. and L.N.; data curation, B.M.S. and G.M.; writing—original draft preparation, V.G. and L.N.; writing—review and editing, F.d. and A.D.I.; visualization, G.D.; supervision, L.P. All authors have read and agreed to the published version of the manuscript.

Funding: This research received no external funding.

Institutional Review Board Statement: Not applicable.

Informed Consent Statement: Not applicable.

Data Availability Statement: Please contact the corresponding author.

Conflicts of Interest: The authors declare no conflict of interest.

References

1. Ngan, P.; Moon, W. Evolution of Class III Treatment in Orthodontics. *Am. J. Orthod. Dentofacial Orthop.* **2015**, *148*, 22–36. [CrossRef]
2. Duggal, R.; Mathur, V.; Parkash, H.; Jena, A. Class—III Malocclusion: Genetics or Environment? A Twins Study. *J. Indian Soc. Pedod. Prev. Dent.* **2005**, *23*, 27. [CrossRef] [PubMed]
3. Adina, S.; Dipalma, G.; Bordea, I.R.; Lucaciu, O.; Feurdean, C.; Inchingolo, A.D.; Septimiu, R.; Malcangi, G.; Cantore, S.; Martin, D.; et al. Orthopedic Joint Stability Influences Growth and Maxillary Development: Clinical Aspects. *J. Biol. Regul. Homeost. Agents* **2020**, *34*, 747–756. [CrossRef]
4. Al-Mozany, S.A.; Dalci, O.; Almuzian, M.; Gonzalez, C.; Tarraf, N.E.; Ali Darendeliler, M. A Novel Method for Treatment of Class III Malocclusion in Growing Patients. *Prog. Orthod.* **2017**, *18*, 40. [CrossRef]
5. Di Venere, D.; Nardi, G.M.; Lacarbonara, V.; Laforgia, A.; Stefanachi, G.; Corsalini, M.; Grassi, F.R.; Rapone, B.; Pettini, F. Early mandibular canine-lateral incisor transposition: Case Report. *Oral Implantol.* **2017**, *10*, 181–189. [CrossRef] [PubMed]

6. Di Venere, D.; Corsalini, M.; Nardi, G.M.; Laforgia, A.; Grassi, F.R.; Rapone, B.; Pettini, F. Obstructive site localization in patients with Obstructive Sleep Apnea Syndrome: A comparison between otolaryngologic data and cephalometric values. *Oral Implantol.* **2017**, *10*, 295–310. [CrossRef] [PubMed]
7. Di Venere, D.; Pettini, F.; Nardi, G.M.; Laforgia, A.; Stefanachi, G.; Notaro, V.; Rapone, B.; Grassi, F.R.; Corsalini, M. Correlation between parodontal indexes and orthodontic retainers: Prospective study in a group of 16 patients. *Oral Implantol.* **2017**, *10*, 78–86. [CrossRef]
8. Cantore, S.; Ballini, A.; Farronato, D.; Malcangi, G.; Dipalma, G.; Assandri, F.; Garagiola, U.; Inchingolo, F.; De Vito, D.; Cirulli, N. Evaluation of an oral appliance in patients with mild to moderate obstructive sleep apnea syndrome intolerant to continuous positive airway pressure use: Preliminary results. *Int. J. Immunopathol. Pharmacol.* **2016**, *29*, 267–273. [CrossRef]
9. Dimonte, M.; Inchingolo, F.; Minonne, A.; Arditi, G.; Dipalma, G. Bone SPECT in management of mandibular condyle hyperplasia. Report of a case and review of literature. *Minerva Stomatol.* **2004**, *53*, 281–285.
10. Sirbu, A.A.; Bordea, R.; Lucaciu, O.; Braitoru, C.; Szuhanek, C.; Campian, R. 3D Printed Splints an Innovative Method to Treat Temporomandibular Joint Pathology. *Rev. Chim.* **2018**, *69*, 3087–3089. [CrossRef]
11. Laudadio, C.; Inchingolo, A.D.; Malcangi, G.; Limongelli, L.; Marinelli, G.; Coloccia, G.; Montenegro, V.; Patano, A.; Inchingolo, F.; Bordea, I.R.; et al. Management of Anterior Open-Bite in the Deciduous, Mixed and Permanent Dentition Stage: A Descriptive Review. *J. Biol. Regul. Homeost. Agents* **2021**, *35*, 271–281. [CrossRef] [PubMed]
12. Coloccia, G.; Inchingolo, A.D.; Inchingolo, A.M.; Malcangi, G.; Montenegro, V.; Patano, A.; Marinelli, G.; Laudadio, C.; Limongelli, L.; Di Venere, D.; et al. Effectiveness of Dental and Maxillary Transverse Changes in Tooth-Borne, Bone-Borne, and Hybrid Palatal Expansion through Cone-Beam Tomography: A Systematic Review of the Literature. *Medicina* **2021**, *57*, 288. [CrossRef] [PubMed]
13. Patano, A.; Cirulli, N.; Beretta, M.; Plantamura, P.; Inchingolo, A.D.; Inchingolo, A.M.; Bordea, I.R.; Malcangi, G.; Marinelli, G.; Scarano, A.; et al. Education Technology in Orthodontics and Paediatric Dentistry during the COVID-19 Pandemic: A Systematic Review. *Int. J. Environ. Res. Public. Health* **2021**, *18*, 6056. [CrossRef] [PubMed]
14. Montenegro, V.; Inchingolo, A.D.; Malcangi, G.; Limongelli, L.; Marinelli, G.; Coloccia, G.; Laudadio, C.; Patano, A.; Inchingolo, F.; Bordea, I.R.; et al. Compliance of Children with Removable Functional Appliance with Microchip Integrated during Covid-19 Pandemic: A Systematic Review. *J. Biol. Regul. Homeost. Agents* **2021**, *35*, 365–377. [CrossRef]
15. Almuzian, M.; Almukhtar, A.; Ulhaq, A.; Alharbi, F.; Darendeliler, M.A. 3D Effects of a Bone-Anchored Intra-Oral Protraction in Treating Class III Growing Patient: A Pilot Study. *Prog. Orthod.* **2019**, *20*, 37. [CrossRef]
16. Grassia, V.; d'Apuzzo, F.; DiStasio, D.; Jamilian, A.; Lucchese, A.; Perillo, L. Upper and Lower Arch Changes after Mixed Palatal Expansion Protocol. *Eur. J. Paediatr. Dent.* **2014**, *15*, 375–380.
17. Page, M.J.; McKenzie, J.E.; Bossuyt, P.M.; Boutron, I.; Hoffmann, T.C.; Mulrow, C.D.; Shamseer, L.; Tetzlaff, J.M.; Akl, E.A.; Brennan, S.E.; et al. The PRISMA 2020 statement: An updated guideline for reporting systematic reviews. *BMJ* **2021**, *71*, 372. [CrossRef]
18. Alzabibi, B.A.; Burhan, A.S.; Hajeer, M.Y.; Nawaya, F.R. Short-term effects of the orthodontic removable traction appliance in the treatment of skeletal Class III malocclusion: A randomized controlled trial. *Dent. Med. Probl.* **2021**, *58*, 163–172. [CrossRef]
19. Fatima, F.; Jeelani, W.; Ahmed, M. Current trends in craniofacial distraction: A literature review. *Dent. Med. Probl.* **2020**, *57*, 441–448. [CrossRef]
20. Fabozzi, F.F.; Nucci, L.; Correra, A.; d'Apuzzo, F.; Franchi, L.; Perillo, L. Comparison of Two Protocols for Early Treatment of Dentoskeletal Class III Malocclusion: Modified SEC III versus RME/FM. *Orthod. Craniofac. Res.* **2021**, *24*, 344–350. [CrossRef]
21. Inchingolo, A.D.; Patano, A.; Coloccia, G.; Ceci, S.; Inchingolo, A.M.; Marinelli, G.; Malcangi, G.; Montenegro, V.; Laudadio, C.; Palmieri, G.; et al. Genetic Pattern, Orthodontic and Surgical Management of Multiple Supplementary Impacted Teeth in a Rare, Cleidocranial Dysplasia Patient: A Case Report. *Medicina* **2021**, *57*, 1350. [CrossRef] [PubMed]
22. Giugliano, D.; d'Apuzzo, F.; Majorana, A.; Campus, G.; Nucci, F.; Flores-Mir, C.; Perillo, L. Influence of occlusal characteristics, food intake and oral hygiene habits on dental caries in adolescents: A cross-sectional study. *Eur. J. Paediatr. Dent.* **2018**, *19*, 95–100. [CrossRef] [PubMed]
23. Franchi, L.; Baccetti, T.; McNamara, J.A. Postpubertal Assessment of Treatment Timing for Maxillary Expansion and Protraction Therapy Followed by Fixed Appliances. *Am. J. Orthod. Dentofacial Orthop.* **2004**, *126*, 555–568. [CrossRef] [PubMed]
24. Patianna, A.G.; Ballini, A.; Meneghello, M.; Cantore, S.; Inchingolo, A.M.; Dipalma, G.; Inchingolo, A.D.; Inchingolo, F.; Malcangi, G.; Lucchese, A.; et al. Comparison of conventional orthognathic surgery and "surgery-first" protocol: A new weapon against time. *J. Biol. Regul. Homeost. Agents* **2019**, *33*, 59–67. [PubMed]
25. Quaglia, E.; Moscufo, L.; Corsalini, M.; Coscia, D.; Sportelli, P.; Cantatore, F.; De Rinaldis, C.; Rapone, B.; Carossa, M.; Carossa, S. Polyamide vs silk sutures in the healing of postextraction sockets: A split mouth study. *Oral Implantol.* **2018**, *11*, 115–120.
26. Rapone, B.; Ferrara, E.; Corsalini, M.; Converti, I.; Grassi, F.R.; Santacroce, L.; Topi, S.; Gnoni, A.; Scacco, S.; Scarano, A.; et al. The Effect of Gaseous Ozone Therapy in Conjunction with Periodontal Treatment on Glycated Hemoglobin Level in Subjects with Type 2 Diabetes Mellitus: An Unmasked Randomized Controlled Trial. *Int. J. Environ. Res. Public Health* **2020**, *17*, 54675. [CrossRef]
27. Farronato, M.; Farronato, D.; Inchingolo, F.; Grassi, L.; Lanteri, V.; Maspero, C. Evaluation of Dental Surface after De-Bonding Orthodontic Bracket Bonded with a Novel Fluorescent Composite: In Vitro Comparative Study. *Appl. Sci.* **2021**, *11*, 6354. [CrossRef]

28. Inchingolo, F.; Tatullo, M.; Marrelli, M.; Inchingolo, A.M.; Tarullo, A.; Inchingolo, A.D.; Dipalma, G.; Brunetti, S.P.; Tarullo, A.; Cagiano, R. Combined Occlusal and Pharmacological Therapy in the Treatment of Temporo-Mandibular Disorders. *Eur. Rev. Med. Pharmacol. Sci.* **2011**, *15*, 1296–1300.
29. Wilmes, B.; Nienkemper, M.; Drescher, D. Application and Effectiveness of a Mini-Implant- and Tooth-Borne Rapid Palatal Expansion Device: The Hybrid Hyrax. *World J. Orthod.* **2010**, *11*, 323–330.
30. Grassi, F.R.; Grassi, R.; Rapone, B.; Gianfranco, A.; Balena, A.; Kalemaj, Z. Dimensional changes of buccal bone plate in immediate implants inserted through open flap, open flap and bone grafting, and flapless technique. A CBCT randomized controlled clinical trial. *Clin Oral Implants Res.* **2019**, *30*, 1155–1164. [CrossRef]
31. Rapone, B.; Corsalini, M.; Converti, I.; Loverro, M.T.; Gnoni, A.; Trerotoli, P.; Ferrara, E. Does Periodontal Inflammation Affect Type 1 Diabetes in Childhood and Adolescence? A Meta-Analysis. *Front. Endocrinol.* **2020**, *11*, 278. [CrossRef] [PubMed]
32. Ballini, A.; Cantore, S.; Scacco, S.; Perillo, L.; Scarano, A.; Aityan, S.K.; Contaldo, M.; Nguyen, K.C.; Santacroce, L.; Syed, J.; et al. A comparative study on different stemness gene expression between dental pulp stem cells vs. dental bud stem cells. *Eur. Rev. Med. Pharmacol. Sci.* **2019**, *23*, 1626–1633. [PubMed]
33. Grassi, F.R.; Rapone, B.; Scarano Catanzaro, F.; Corsalini, M.; Kalemaj, Z. Effectiveness of computer-assisted anesthetic delivery system (STA™) in dental implant surgery: A prospective study. *Oral Implantol.* **2017**, *10*, 381–389. [CrossRef] [PubMed]
34. Corsalini, M.; Di Venere, D.; Carossa, M.; Ripa, M.; Sportelli, P.; Cantatore, F.; De Rinaldis, C.; Di Santantonio, G.; Lenoci, G.; Barile, G.; et al. Comparative clinical study between zirconium-ceramic and metal-ceramic fixed rehabilitations. *Oral Implantol.* **2018**, *11*, 150–160.
35. Ballini, A.; Cantore, S.; Fotopoulou, E.A.; Georgakopoulos, I.P.; Athanasiou, E.; Bellos, D.; Paduanelli, G.; Saini, R.; Dipalma, G.; Inchingolo, F. Combined sea salt-based oral rinse with xylitol in orthodontic patients: Clinical and microbiological study. *J. Biol. Regul. Homeost. Agents* **2019**, *33*, 263–268.
36. Rapone, B.; Ferrara, E.; Santacroce, L.; Cesarano, F.; Arazzi, M.; Di Liberato, L.; Scacco, S.; Grassi, R.; Grassi, F.R.; Gnoni, A.; et al. Periodontal Microbiological Status Influences the Occurrence of Cyclosporine-A and Tacrolimus- Induced Gingival Overgrowth. *Antibiotics* **2019**, *8*, 124. [CrossRef]
37. Corsalini, M.; Di Venere, D.; Sportelli, P.; Magazzino, D.; Ripa, M.; Cantatore, F.; Cagnetta, C.; De Rinaldis, C.; Montemurro, N.; De Giacomo, A.; et al. Evaluation of prosthetic quality and masticatory efficiency in patients with total removable prosthesis: Study of 12 cases. *Oral Implantol.* **2018**, *11*, 230–240.
38. Cantore, S.; Ballini, A.; De Vito, D.; Martelli, F.S.; Georgakopoulos, I.; Almasri, M.; Dibello, V.; Altini, V.; Farronato, G.; Dipalma, G.; et al. Characterization of human apical papilla-derived stem cells. *J. Biol. Regul. Homeost. Agents* **2017**, *31*, 901–910.
39. Marinelli, G.; Inchingolo, A.D.; Inchingolo, A.M.; Malcangi, G.; Limongelli, L.; Montenegro, V.; Coloccia, G.; Laudadio, C.; Patano, A.; Inchingolo, F.; et al. White spot lesions in orthodontics: Prevention and treatment. A descriptive review. *J. Biol. Regul. Homeost. Agents* **2021**, *35*, 227–240.
40. Cirulli, N.; Ballini, A.; Cantore, S.; Farronato, D.; Inchingolo, F.; Dipalma, G.; Gatto, M.R.; Alessandri Bonetti, G. Mixed dentition space analysis of a southern italian population: New regression equations for unerupted teeth. *J. Biol. Regul. Homeost. Agents* **2015**, *29*, 515–520.
41. Cevidanes, L.; Baccetti, T.; Franchi, L.; McNamara, J.A.; De Clerck, H. Comparison of Two Protocols for Maxillary Protraction: Bone Anchors versus Face Mask with Rapid Maxillary Expansion. *Angle Orthod.* **2010**, *80*, 799–806. [CrossRef] [PubMed]
42. Heymann, G.C.; Cevidanes, L.; Cornelis, M.; De Clerck, H.J.; Tulloch, J.F.C. Three-Dimensional Analysis of Maxillary Protraction with Intermaxillary Elastics to Miniplates. *Am. J. Orthod. Dentofacial Orthop.* **2010**, *137*, 274–284. [CrossRef] [PubMed]
43. Scarano, A.; Inchingolo, F.; Rapone, B.; Festa, F.; Tari, S.R.; Lorusso, F. Protective Face Masks: Effect on the Oxygenation and Heart Rate Status of Oral Surgeons during Surgery. *Int. J. Environ. Res. Public Health* **2021**, *18*, 2363. [CrossRef] [PubMed]
44. Lorusso, F.; Noumbissi, S.; Inchingolo, F.; Rapone, B.; Khater, A.G.A.; Scarano, A. Scientific Trends in Clinical Research on Zirconia Dental Implants: A Bibliometric Review. *Materials* **2020**, *13*, 5534. [CrossRef] [PubMed]
45. Bordea, I.; Sîrbu, A.; Lucaciu, O.; Ilea, A.; Câmpian, R.; Todea, D.; Alexescu, T.; Aluaș, M.; Budin, C.; Pop, A. Microleakage—The Main Culprit in Bracket Bond Failure? *J. Mind Med. Sci.* **2019**, *6*, 86–94. [CrossRef]
46. Moon, W.; Wu, K.W.; MacGinnis, M.; Sung, J.; Chu, H.; Youssef, G.; Machado, A. The Efficacy of Maxillary Protraction Protocols with the Micro-Implant-Assisted Rapid Palatal Expander (MARPE) and the Novel N2 Mini-Implant—a Finite Element Study. *Prog. Orthod.* **2015**, *16*, 16. [CrossRef]
47. Ottawa Hospital Research Institute. Available online: http://www.ohri.ca/programs/clinical_epidemiology/oxford.asp (accessed on 26 January 2022).
48. Montinaro, F.; Nucci, L.; Carfora, M.; d'Apuzzo, F.; Franchi, L.; Perillo, L. Modified SEC III Protocol: Vertical Control Related to Patients' Compliance with the Chincup. *Eur. J. Orthod.* **2021**, *43*, 80–85. [CrossRef]
49. Maino, G.; Turci, Y.; Arreghini, A.; Paoletto, E.; Siciliani, G.; Lombardo, L. Skeletal and Dentoalveolar Effects of Hybrid Rapid Palatal Expansion and Facemask Treatment in Growing Skeletal Class III Patients. *Am. J. Orthod. Dentofacial Orthop.* **2018**, *153*, 262–268. [CrossRef]
50. Hourfar, J.; Kinzinger, G.S.M.; Ludwig, B.; Spindler, J.; Lisson, J.A. Differential Treatment Effects of Two Anchorage Systems for Rapid Maxillary Expansion: A Retrospective Cephalometric Study. *J. Orofac. Orthop. Fortschr. Kieferorthopädie* **2016**, *77*, 314–324. [CrossRef]

51. Nienkemper, M.; Wilmes, B.; Franchi, L.; Drescher, D. Effectiveness of Maxillary Protraction Using a Hybrid Hyrax-Facemask Combination: A Controlled Clinical Study. *Angle Orthod.* **2015**, *85*, 764–770. [CrossRef]
52. Marra, P.M.; Nucci, L.; Abdolreza, J.; Perillo, L.; Itro, A.; Grassia, V. Odontoma in a young and anxious patient associated with unerupted permanent mandibular cuspid: A case report. *J. Int. Oral Health* **2020**, *12*, 182–186. [CrossRef]
53. Willmann, J.H.; Nienkemper, M.; Tarraf, N.E.; Wilmes, B.; Drescher, D. Early Class III Treatment with Hybrid-Hyrax -Facemask in Comparison to Hybrid-Hyrax-Mentoplate—Skeletal and Dental Outcomes. *Prog. Orthod.* **2018**, *19*, 42. [CrossRef] [PubMed]
54. Ngan, P.; Wilmes, B.; Drescher, D.; Martin, C.; Weaver, B.; Gunel, E. Comparison of Two Maxillary Protraction Protocols: Tooth-Borne versus Bone-Anchored Protraction Facemask Treatment. *Prog. Orthod.* **2015**, *16*, 26. [CrossRef] [PubMed]
55. Seiryu, M.; Ida, H.; Mayama, A.; Sasaki, S.; Sasaki, S.; Deguchi, T.; Takano-Yamamoto, T. A Comparative Assessment of Orthodontic Treatment Outcomes of Mild Skeletal Class III Malocclusion Between Facemask and Facemask in Combination with a Miniscrew For Anchorage in Growing Patients: A Single-Center, Prospective Randomized Controlled Trial. *Angle Orthod.* **2020**, *90*, 3–12. [CrossRef]
56. Dekel, E.; Nucci, L.; Weill, T.; Flores-Mir, C.; Becker, A.; Perillo, L.; Chaushu, S. Impaction of Maxillary Canines and Its Effect on the Position of Adjacent Teeth and Canine Development: A Cone-Beam Computed Tomography Study. *Am. J. Orthod. Dentofacial Orthop.* **2021**, *159*, e135–e147. [CrossRef]
57. Eslami, S.; Faber, J.; Fateh, A.; Sheikholaemmeh, F.; Grassia, V.; Jamilian, A. Treatment Decision in Adult Patients with Class III Malocclusion: Surgery versus Orthodontics. *Prog. Orthod.* **2018**, *19*, 28. [CrossRef]
58. Clemente, R.; Contardo, L.; Greco, C.; Di Lenarda, R.; Perinetti, G. Class III Treatment with Skeletal and Dental Anchorage: A Review of Comparative Effects. *BioMed Res. Int.* **2018**, *2018*. [CrossRef]
59. Luchian, I.; Moscalu, M.; Goriuc, A.; Nucci, L.; Tatarciuc, M.; Martu, I.; Covasa, M. Using Salivary MMP-9 to Successfully Quantify Periodontal Inflammation during Orthodontic Treatment. *J. Clin. Med.* **2021**, *10*, 379. [CrossRef]
60. De Felice, M.E.; Nucci, L.; Fiori, A.; Flores-Mir, C.; Perillo, L.; Grassia, V. Accuracy of interproximal enamel reduction during clear aligner treatment. *Prog. Orthod.* **2020**, *21*, 28. [CrossRef]
61. Inchingolo, A.D.; Patano, A.; Coloccia, G.; Ceci, S.; Inchingolo, A.M.; Marinelli, G.; Malcangi, G.; Di Pede, C.; Garibaldi, M.; Ciocia, A.M.; et al. Treatment of Class III Malocclusion and Anterior Crossbite with Aligners: A Case Report. *Medicina* **2022**, *58*, 603. [CrossRef]

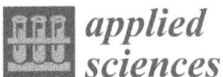

Case Report

Impacted Central Incisors in the Upper Jaw in an Adolescent Patient: Orthodontic-Surgical Treatment—A Case Report

Giuseppina Malcangi [1,*,†], Alessio Danilo Inchingolo [1,*,†], Assunta Patano [1], Giovanni Coloccia [1], Sabino Ceci [1], Mariagrazia Garibaldi [1], Angelo Michele Inchingolo [1], Fabio Piras [1], Filippo Cardarelli [1], Vito Settanni [1], Biagio Rapone [1], Alberto Corriero [1], Antonio Mancini [1], Massimo Corsalini [1], Ludovica Nucci [2], Ioana Roxana Bordea [3,*], Felice Lorusso [4,*], Antonio Scarano [4]T, Delia Giovanniello [5], Gianna Dipalma [1], Vito Marino Posa [6], Daniela Di Venere [1,‡] and Francesco Inchingolo [1,‡]

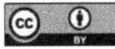

Citation: Malcangi, G.; Inchingolo, A.D.; Patano, A.; Coloccia, G.; Ceci, S.; Garibaldi, M.; Inchingolo, A.M.; Piras, F.; Cardarelli, F.; Settanni, V.; et al. Impacted Central Incisors in the Upper Jaw in an Adolescent Patient: Orthodontic-Surgical Treatment—A Case Report. *Appl. Sci.* **2022**, *12*, 2657. https://doi.org/10.3390/app12052657

Academic Editor: Andrea Scribante

Received: 10 February 2022
Accepted: 2 March 2022
Published: 4 March 2022

Publisher's Note: MDPI stays neutral with regard to jurisdictional claims in published maps and institutional affiliations.

Copyright: © 2022 by the authors. Licensee MDPI, Basel, Switzerland. This article is an open access article distributed under the terms and conditions of the Creative Commons Attribution (CC BY) license (https://creativecommons.org/licenses/by/4.0/).

[1] Department of Interdisciplinary Medicine, University of Bari Aldo Moro, 70124 Bari, Italy; assuntapatano@gmail.com (A.P.); giovanni.coloccia@gmail.com (G.C.); s.ceci@studenti.uniba.it (S.C.); mgr.garibaldi@libero.it (M.G.); angeloinchingolo@gmail.com (A.M.I.); dott.fabio.piras@gmail.com (F.P.); drfilippocardarelli@libero.it (F.C.); v.settanni@libero.it (V.S.); biagiorapone79@gmail.com (B.R.); alberto.corriero@gmail.com (A.C.); dr.antonio.mancini@gmail.com (A.M.); massimo.corsalini@uniba.it (M.C.); giannadipalma@tiscali.it (G.D.); daniela.divenere@uniba.it (D.D.V.); francesco.inchingolo@uniba.it (F.I.)
[2] Multidisciplinary Department of Medical-Surgical and Dental Specialties, University of Campania Luigi Vanvitelli, 80138 Naples, Italy; ludovica.nucci@unicampania.it
[3] Department of Oral Rehabilitation, Faculty of Dentistry, Iuliu Hațieganu University of Medicine and Pharmacy, 400012 Cluj-Napoca, Romania
[4] Department of Innovative Technologies in Medicine and Dentistry, University of Chieti-Pescara, 66100 Chieti, Italy; ascarano@unich.it
[5] Department of Toracic Surgery, Hospital San Camillo Forlanini, 00152 Rome, Italy; giovanniellodelia@gmail.com
[6] Polymedical Clinic Peucezia, 70023 Gioia del Colle, Italy; vitomarinoposa@gmail.com
* Correspondence: giuseppinamalcangi@libero.it (G.M.); ad.inchingolo@libero.it (A.D.I.); roxana.bordea@ymail.com (I.R.B.); felice.lorusso@unich.it (F.L.)
† These authors contributed equally to this work as first authors.
‡ These authors contributed equally to this work as last authors.

Abstract: The inclusion of both maxillary permanent central incisors is uncommon. This condition compromises face aesthetics, phonation and masticatory function. Therefore, early diagnosis is essential to avoid complications and failures. There are various reasons for inclusion, but supernumerary teeth are the leading cause. Early causes of removal and rapid expansion of the palate determine a high probability of success with the spontaneous eruption of the impacted elements. However, it is often necessary to proceed with a surgical–orthodontic treatment. The inclination of teeth in relation to the midline and the root maturation degree determine prognosis and therapeutic timing. In this case report, the orthopantomogram (OPG) X-ray of a 9-year-old boy revealed two impacted supernumerary teeth in the anterior maxillary region, preventing the eruption of the permanent upper central incisors. The impacted supernumerary teeth were surgically removed at different times. A straight wire multibrackets technique associated with a fixed palatal appliance was used. The palatal appliance featured an osteomucous resin support at the level of the retroincisal papilla. Subsequently, surgical exposure was carried out using the closed eruption technique and elastic traction, bringing 11 and 21 back into the arch.

Keywords: impacted incisors; supernumeraries; dental inclusion; orthodontic treatment; closed-eruption surgical technique; guided eruption; surgical exposure

1. Introduction

Eruption anomalies are classified into position-related disorders (ectopic eruption and transpositions) and timing-related disorders (premature eruption, delayed eruption or impaction). These anomalies are also linked to age, sex, race or ethnicity. Both root developmental staging and patient age are used as criteria to diagnose prematurity or delayed eruption [1–3].

Eruption disorders are more frequent in the upper arch (69.9%) and the area of the incisors (51.2%). Furthermore, in 20.5% of cases, first-degree relatives present the same issue [4,5].

Impaction of the upper central incisors is a rare occurrence (0.06–0.12%), more frequent in men than in women (1.5:1) [4,6].

Traumatic and obstructive causes are the main factors related to impacted teeth [7].

Dental trauma at a young age could damage the non-erupted permanent tooth germ, reduce root development, and change eruption direction. This can lead to dilacerated tooth development with a high risk of uneruption without an orthognathic–surgical therapy [8,9].

Necrosis or ankylosis of a deciduous tooth and the simultaneous presence of systemic pathologies (endocrine diseases, cleidocranial dysostosis) can also determine dental inclusions [10,11].

The main obstructive causes are: odontomas (complex or compound); follicular cysts; thick mucosa; bone tissue formed as a result of the early extraction of a deciduous tooth; and supernumerary teeth [8].

The most common obstructive cause is determined by supernumerary teeth (ST), 77.8% of the ST are found in the maxilla, and 97.2% are in the frontal region. In the anterior maxillary region, the presence of one or more supernumerary teeth along the midline (1.5% to 3.5%) hinders the eruption of the incisors (28% to 60%) [5,12–16].

Although the percentage of upper central incisors uneruption or inclusion is low, its occurrence causes an aesthetic, phonetic and functional discomfort to the patient, arousing parents' concern [7,14].

Parents of an impacted incisor affected child are usually motivated to seek an earlier orthodontic treatment than parents of a child with other orthodontic problems [8,17,18].

The diagnosis of impacted incisors is based on the clinical examination that ascertains and identifies the retained tooth. Palpating the corresponding alveolar area (both palatal and vestibular), a painless, incompressible, fibromucosal bump can be appreciated [19].

The diagnosis needs to be completed by radiological examinations:

(1) Intraoral X-rays with periapical and occlusal projections confirm the presence, position and/or anomaly of the retained maxillary incisors and any underlying developmental anomaly or pathology. The buccolingual position of the non-erupted tooth can be localized using horizontal or vertical parallax.
(2) Ortopanthomography X-ray (OPG X-ray) to evaluate the problem in relation to the entire arch, adjacent tooth and the staging of the eruption of the other dental elements.
(3) Latero-Lateral Teleradiography (LLT) of the head with cephalometric trace to assess the height and inclination of the crown and root of the impacted tooth.
(4) Cone-Beam Computed Tomography (CBCT) for a three-dimensional evaluation of impacted elements and surrounding structures.

All these data allow us to correctly plan the treatment and the optimal direction of traction in order to have a correct extrusion of the impacted tooth with adequate periodontal support [19–21].

Early treatment is essential because the non-erupted maxillary central incisor can cause various issues:

(1) Compromission of the aesthetic aspect, phonation and alveolar ridge formation.
(2) Increase of adjacent teeth tip, reducing the space for the non-erupted incisor.
(3) Alteration of the eruptive path (deviation and delay) of the ipsilateral canine [10].

The treatment options for impacted incisors include:

(1) Extraction of the impacted tooth followed by a prosthetic rehabilitation [22–24];
(2) Extraction and repositioning of the lateral incisor in place of the central incisor with mesial canine and premolar movement, then coronoplasty;

(3) Surgical-orthodontic recovery of the incisor [25,26].

Most of the patients requiring impacted central incisors treatment are less than 12 years old; for this reason, the prosthetic solution is not suitable. The extraction of the affected tooth would lead to a severe loss of alveolar bone, compromising the future insertion of an implant [18]. On the other side, the surgical–orthodontic solution allows complete alignment of natural teeth and does not require the creation of a prosthesis [25,26].

Treatment success rates depend on several factors:

(1) The angle between impacted incisor and midline (if greater than 20 degrees, there are greater difficulties in treatment and a worse prognosis);
(2) The level of the crown of the impacted tooth compared to the eruptive age;
(3) The distance of the impacted incisor from the occlusal plane [8,25,27,28].

A study has verified that performing a rapid expansion with a Rapid Maxillary Expander (RME) immediately after the obstacle removal leads to an 82% chance of problem resolution with the eruption of the impacted element after 6–7 months from the obstacle removal, while without applying the RME, the percentages are reduced by 39% [25,29,30].

Several surgical techniques are commonly used to expose the maxillary teeth. One technique is the apical repositioning flap. It consists of the apical repositioning of a raised full-thickness-flap above the included tooth, leaving the element uncovered. Another technique is the closed eruption. It involves lifting a full-thickness flap, fixing an orthodontic bracket on the tooth surface, and then completely covering the tooth and bracket with tissue. These techniques offer some advantages when pulling impacted teeth [10,31,32].

The apically repositioned flap technique allows prompt reattachment of the bracket if unintentional detachment occurs. However, the closed eruption technique provides the most aesthetically pleasing result. This technique is most reliable when considering aesthetic and periodontal health. Vermette et al., recommended using the closed eruption technique when the tooth is in the center of the socket or when it is high, near the nasal spine. In these cases, the periodontal state of the exposed teeth after orthodontic treatment usually revealed an acceptable gingival profile and good adherent gingiva, an increase in bone level on the mesial, vestibular and distal surfaces, requiring no further mucogingival surgery [33].

Since many variables affect the recovery of an included tooth in a child after removing the supernumerary elements or the odontoma, most studies believe orthodontic treatment is necessary rather than waiting for the spontaneous eruption [8,25,34].

The treatment of impacted central incisors requires a different approach, and it is longer and more complicated, with the resolution of extraction with subsequent prosthetic rehabilitation as a valid alternative [35].

According to the latest literature data, the approach for this type of issue is mainly oriented to surgical–orthodontic treatments [36,37].

Undoubtedly, the best treatment choice is conservative, and it requires careful planning and close collaboration between orthodontists, oral surgeons and periodontists. Studies report that the prognosis of orthodontic–surgical treatment of impacted incisors is good, and failures occur when the etiology of the inclusion is dilaceration [36].

The treatment is relatively long, approximately two years, and is influenced by the initial height of the tooth included in the jaw [38].

2. Case Report

A 15-year and 6-months-old patient (F.F.) comes to our attention.

2.1. Clinical History

The patient had previously undergone orthodontic treatment since the age of 9, the presence of persistent deciduous (51 and 61), and two ST were found in areas 11 and 21 preventing their eruption (Figure 1).

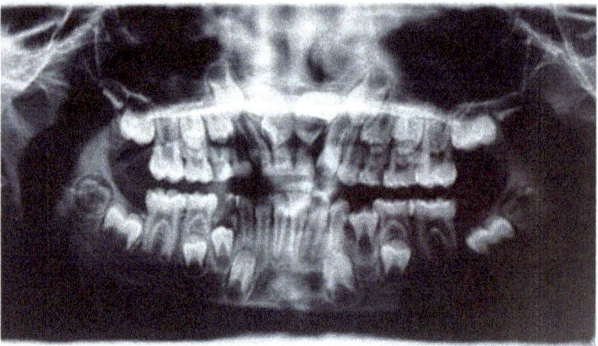

Figure 1. F.F. 9y, OPG X-ray initial clinical evaluation with persistent deciduous 51–61, supernumerary teeth and impacted incisors 11–21.

The two ST were removed at different times (10-years-old and 13-year-old), and a late rapid expansion (14-year-old) was performed without any improvement (Figures 2 and 3).

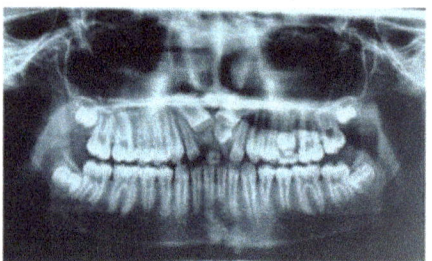

Figure 2. F.F. 13y OPG X-ray presence of one supernumerary tooth and impacted incisors 11–21.

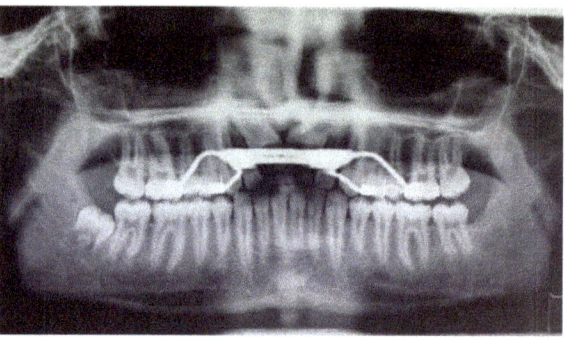

Figure 3. F.F. 14y OPG X-ray after RME.

2.2. Clinical Exams and Diagnosis

Patient in good health. Clinical evaluation revealed the absence of teeth 11 and 21.

The orthodontic situation was re-evaluated with new intraoral photos and X-rays (Figures 4 and 5).

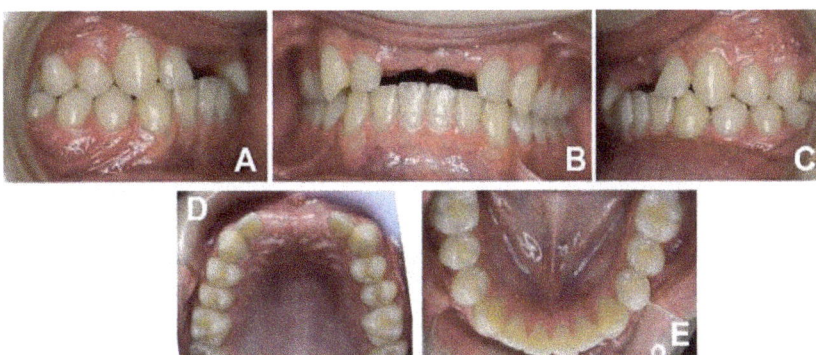

Figure 4. (A–E) F.F. 15y 6m intraoral photos at the beginning of treatment: right (**A**), front (**B**), and left (**C**) view; occlusal upper (**D**), and occlusal lower (**E**) view.

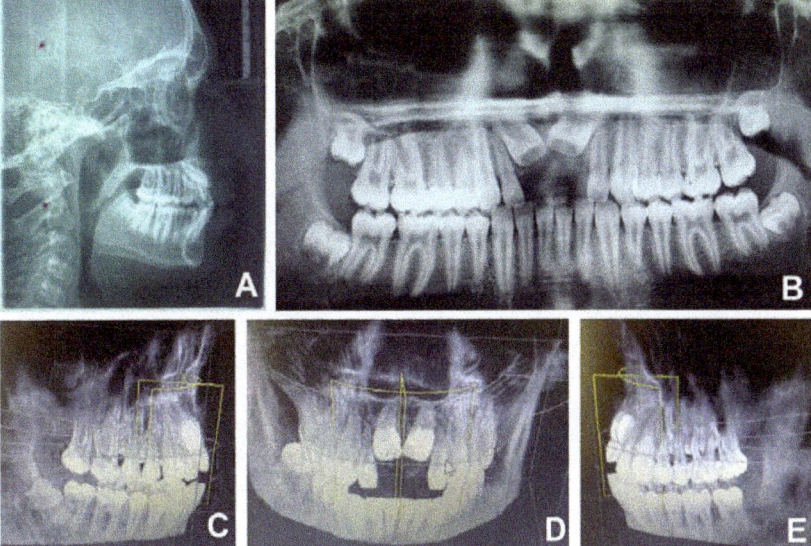

Figure 5. (A–E) F.F. 15y 6m initial radiographic documentation: LLT (**A**), OPG X-ray (**B**), CBCT right (**C**), front (**D**), and left (**E**) view.

The patient had molar and canine class I, dental and skeletal malocclusion, counter-clockwise mandibular growth with a tendency to brachycephalic growth, good transverse dimension arch and slight lower crowding. To confirm the position and relationship with adjacent structures, CBCT was recommended. The position of the two upper incisors was assessable with CBCT and LLT.

The 11 and 21 presented a very apical position (immediately under the anterior nasal spine) and a significant inclination (51.2°) (Figure 6 and Table 1).

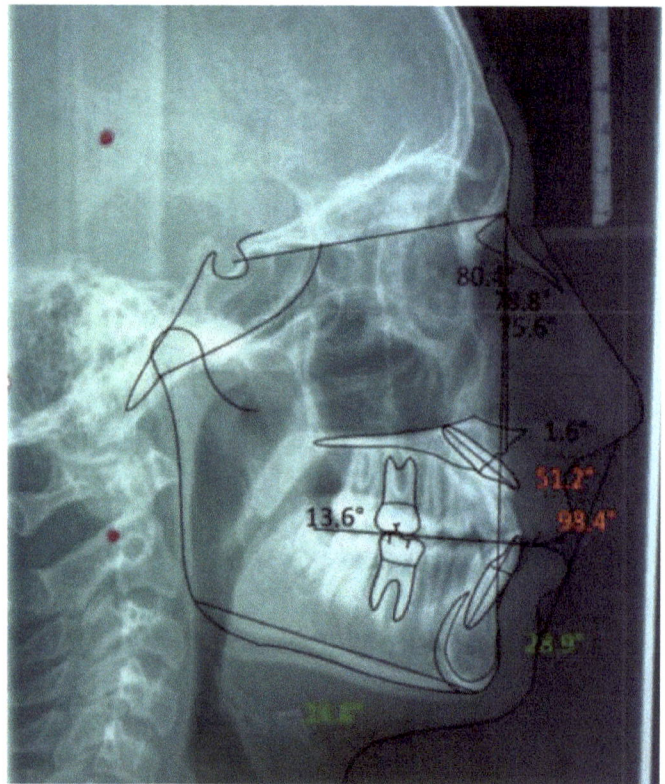

Figure 6. F.F. 15y 6m Steiner's cephalometric tracing.

Table 1. F.F. 15y 6m Steiner's cephalometric analysis.

	Values	Normal
SNA	80.4°	82°+/−2°
SNB	78.8°	80°+/−2°
ANB	1.6°	2°+/−2°
GONIAC ANGLE	116.1°	130°+/−7°
INTERINCISIVE ANGLE	98.4°	131°+/−6°
SUPERIOR INCISOR ANGLE	51.2°	22°+/−2°
INFERIOR INCISOR ANGLE	28.9°	25°+/−2°

The patient wore a removable prosthetic device for aesthetic and functional purposes to replace elements 21 and 11 (Figure 7).

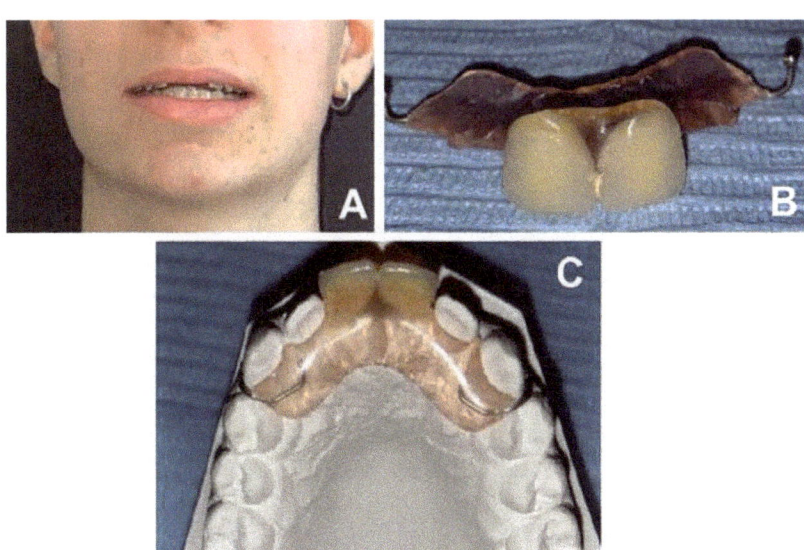

Figure 7. (**A–C**) removable prosthetic device for aesthetic and functional purposes to replace elements 21 and 11: patient frontal smile (**A**); prosthetic device frontal view (**B**); cast model and prosthetic device occlusal view (**C**).

2.3. Therapeutic Plan

An orthodontic–surgical therapy that aimed to pull down the two elements and bring them into a more occlusal position was adopted. Initially, the elements of the upper arch were aligned with a fixed straight-wire multibrackets technique, which also made it possible to apply a pontic in areas 11 and 21, not to compromise the aesthetic and functional aspects of the patient. After osteotomy, a full-thickness flap was made to access the crowns using a scalpel. After dental exposure, two eyelets were bonded, and elastic tractions were applied. The flap was then positioned to cover the teeth and buttons according to the closed eruption technique. On 16 and 26, a fixed palatal appliance was cemented, with supports on 14/24 and a retroincisive papillae osteomucosal resin support. This was done to allow the elements to be pulled without causing unwanted movement of adjacent elements due to the action-reaction effect. The front resin portion was equipped with three loops to allow elastic traction in several directions (Figure 8).

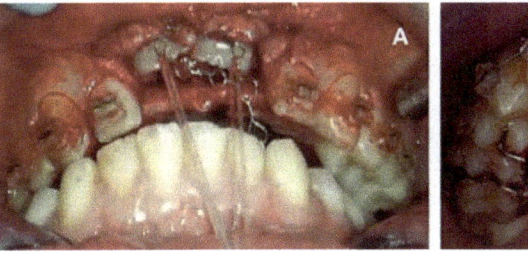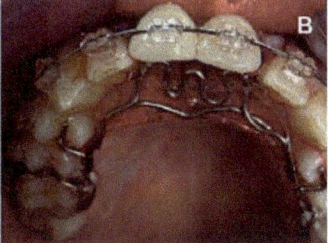

Figure 8. (**A**,**B**) post-operative view before device placement (**A**); fixed palatal appliance with three loops and central incisors pontic (**B**).

After ten months, the upper incisors emerged from the gingiva and reached a more occlusal position. A further diode laser uncovering and modelling of the mucosa was carried out. A 0.019 × 0.025 steel arch was used as anchorage while central incisors were engaged with a 0.014 thermal nickel-titanium (NiTi) arch (Figure 9).

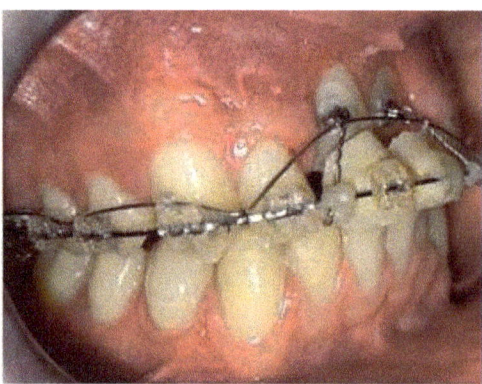

Figure 9. Upper 0.019 × 0.025 steel arch with a 0.014 thermal nickel-titanium.

Subsequently, the prosthetic elements were removed, and the eyelets were replaced with metal brackets. This allowed the extrusion with the 0.014 thermal NiTi arch properly engaged (Figure 10).

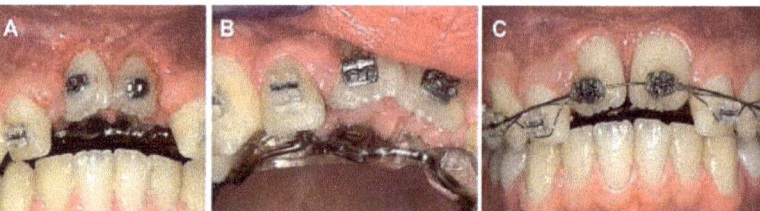

Figure 10. (A–C): Central incisors with eyelets (**A**); central incisors with brackets (**B**); central incisors extrusion with 0.014 thermal NiTi arch properly engaged (**C**).

After three months, the incisors were further extruded and almost aligned with the other elements of the upper arch. Thus, it was possible to engage the 0.014 thermal NiTi base arch. The metal brackets on 11 and 21 have been further replaced with aesthetic twin brackets.

The fixed orthodontic treatment was then also started in the lower arch.

3. Results

After 24 months of treatment (including COVID-19 lockdown periods), 11 and 21 were correctly positioned in the occlusal plane with good bone and periodontal support.

The patient improved the vertical dimension, the upper lip support and the smile aesthetics (Figures 11–13).

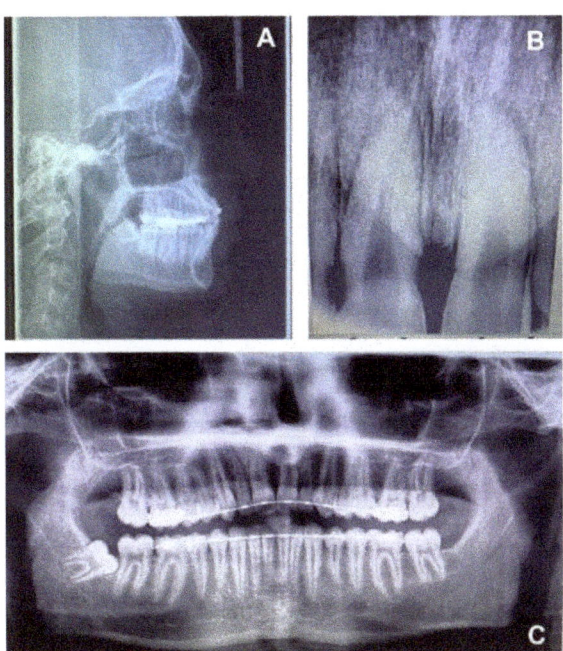

Figure 11. (**A–C**) F.F. 17y 7m final radiographic documentation: LLT (**A**); central incisors intraoral X-ray (**B**); OPG X-ray (**C**).

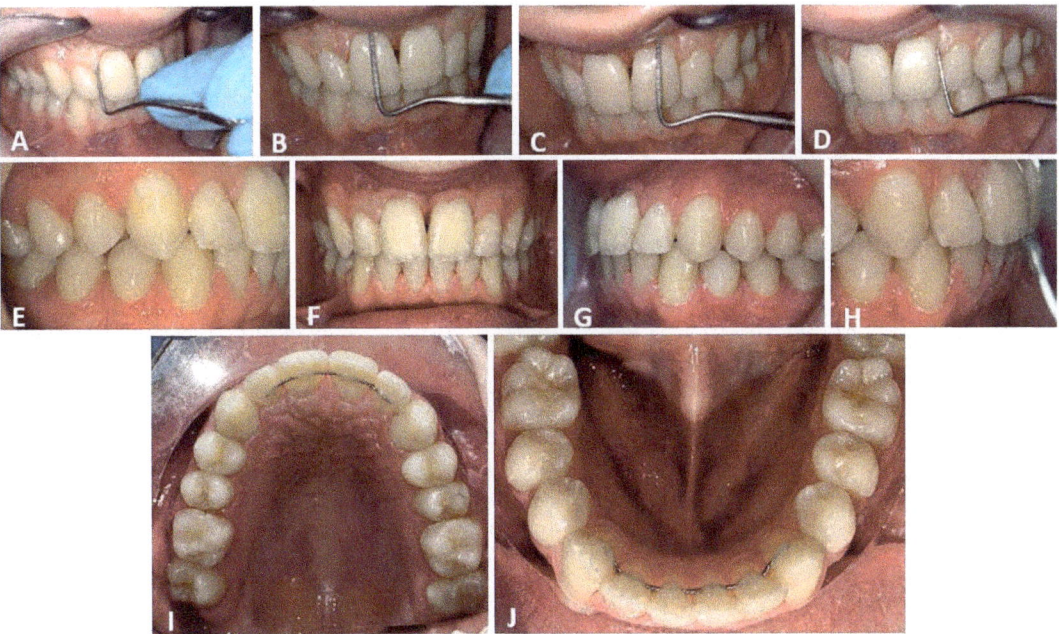

Figure 12. (**A–J**) F.F. 17y 7m final intraoral photos: 11 periodontal probing (**A,B**); 21 periodontal probing (**C,D**); right (**E**), front (**F**) and left (**G**) view; overjet view (**H**); occlusal upper (**I**) and occlusal lower (**J**) view.

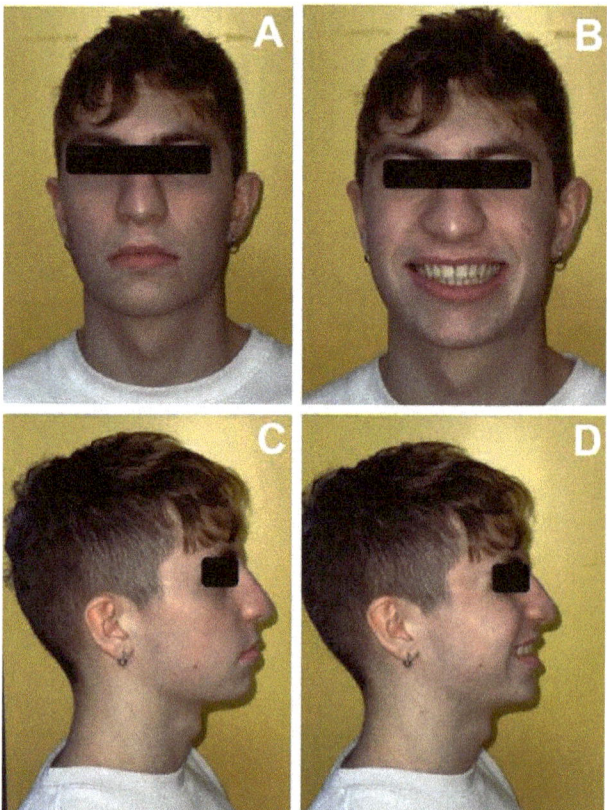

Figure 13. (**A**–**D**) F.F. 17y 7m extraoral photos at the end of the treatment: frontal view closed lips (**A**); frontal view smiling (**B**); facial profile with closed lips (**C**); facial profile smiling (**D**).

4. Discussion

Careful treatment planning of impacted incisors is crucial for a favorable prognosis. It is always multidisciplinary as it requires the intervention of an orthodontist and an oral surgeon [6,16,39].

The choice of the orthodontic–surgical treatment plan with a closed eruption technique and elastic tractions was guided by several factors.

First of all, the patient's age (adolescent) was considered: the patient wore a removable prosthesis that replaced the two missing incisors with significant discomfort [5,40].

Analyzing the patient's clinical history, it emerged that no extrusion movement of the impacted incisors had occurred despite the patient having already removed the two supernumeraries in different periods and had already performed a rapid, although the late, expansion of the palate (14-year-old) [8]. The alternative solution of extraction of impacted teeth and implant therapy was then offered [26].

LLT and CBCT confirmed the unfavorable inclination and height of the crowns. The roots were already wholly developed, so there was no eruptive thrust. Furthermore, no lacerations were reported [33,41]. Parents were also informed of the possibility of treatment failure.

After aligning the upper arch with the straight-wire technique, a full-thickness flap, palatal bone removal and elastic traction with closed eruption were performed. The occlusal plane was stabilized by a molar cemented palatal device, with first upper premolars support arms and an osteo-mucosal support. Otherwise, it could have been affected by the reaction forces caused by extrusion forces [42].

The device choice has been made to allow the patient to have pontics in zone 11–21 during the treatment and not to have discomfort in social life.

During the OPG X-ray and intraoral X-ray examination, good palatal, mesial and distal bone margins were highlighted with more significant resorption on the vestibular side [2,43–47].

The roots were shorter, also in relation to the adjacent lateral incisors. According to the literature, the reabsorption may be due to the initial impediment caused by supernumeraries mobilization and to the orthodontic eruption movement [2].

The treatment lasted 25 months with several periods of inactivation because the patient was treated during the COVID-19 pandemic, including the first lockdown. The elements were correctly positioned on the occlusal plane with an excellent gingival margin [48–50].

Upper and lower restraint with retainers and Essix was adopted [51].

5. Conclusions

An early and accurate diagnosis supported by clinical and radiological examinations, such as OPG X-ray and CBCT, is essential.

It is crucial to evaluate the predictive eruption factors that influence the treatment plan, such as: age of the patient, history, compliance, distance from the occlusal plane, vertical position of unerupted incisors and inclination in relation to the midline.

A complication during the tooth eruption could adversely affect the occlusion development and potentially burden the child's psychological evolution.

The early orthodontic interceptive treatment with obstacle removal and an orthopedic expansion with RME is fundamental.

Elastic tractions with the closed eruption technique for occlusal repositioning is preferred. This approach improves the intraosseous position and the mucogingival condition of the retained tooth.

In general, surgical–orthodontics treatment of impacted incisors has a good chance of success, but it is relatively time-consuming.

It is necessary to inform the patients and their parents of the failure risk and the increased treatment time, especially in the presence of impacted incisors in a very high alveolar position.

Author Contributions: Conceptualization, F.I., A.D.I., A.M.I., D.D.V., G.D., A.S., S.C., G.C., F.L. and A.P.; methodology, A.D.I., M.G., F.C., L.N., A.M., A.C., G.C., F.P., S.C. and M.C.; software, I.R.B., A.P., F.C., S.C., D.G., A.M., F.C. and G.D.; validation, F.I., F.L., F.C., V.S., L.N., G.D., A.D.I., A.M.I. and A.S.; formal analysis, A.M.I., F.L., V.M.P., D.D.V., A.D.I., B.R. and G.M.; investigation, G.M., G.D., A.D.I., F.L., A.M.I., A.P., S.C., A.S. and F.I.; resources, A.M.I., S.C., A.P., G.D., A.D.I., F.I., I.R.B. and G.M.; data curation, G.D., F.C., F.L., M.G., A.M., G.C., M.G., F.I., D.D.V. and G.M.; writing—original draft preparation, A.D.I., A.M.I., G.D., M.G., A.S., F.C., F.L. and F.I.; writing—review and editing, F.I., F.L., D.D.V., G.M., M.G., A.S., V.S. and G.D.; visualization, F.L., A.S. and I.R.B.; supervision, M.G., D.D.V., F.I., A.D.I. and F.L.; project administration, F.I., G.D., G.M., A.P., G.C., S.C. and V.M.P. All authors have read and agreed to the published version of the manuscript.

Funding: This research received no external funding.

Institutional Review Board Statement: The present clinical study was based in the University of Bari (Italy), in full accordance with ethical principles, including the World Medical Association Declaration of Helsinki and the additional requirements of Italian law. Furthermore, the University of Bari, Italy, classified the study to be exempt from ethical review as it carries only negligible risk and involves the use of existing data that contain only non-identifiable data about human beings. The patient signed a written informed consent form.

Informed Consent Statement: Informed consent was obtained from the subjects involved in the study. Written informed consent has been obtained from the patient and his parents to publish this paper.

Data Availability Statement: All experimental data to support the findings of this study are available contacting the corresponding author upon request.

Conflicts of Interest: The authors declare no conflict of interest.

Abbreviations

OPG	Orthopantomography X-ray
RME	Rapid Maxillary Expander
LLT	Latero-Lateral Teleradiography
CBCT	Cone Beam Computed Tomography
ST	Supernumerary teeth
FF	Patient name

References

1. Huber, K.; Suri, L.; Taneja, P. Eruption Disturbances of the Maxillary Incisors: A Literature Review. *J. Clin. Pediatric Dent.* **2008**, *32*, 221–230. [CrossRef] [PubMed]
2. Žarovienė, A.; Grinkevičienė, D.; Trakinienė, G.; Smailienė, D. Post-Treatment Status of Impacted Maxillary Central Incisors Following Surgical-Orthodontic Treatment: A Systematic Review. *Medicina* **2021**, *57*, 783. [CrossRef] [PubMed]
3. Cirulli, N.; Ballini, A.; Cantore, S.; Farronato, D.; Inchingolo, F.; Dipalma, G.; Gatto, M.R.; Alessandri Bonetti, G. Mixed Dentition Space Analysis of A Southern Italian Population: New Regression Equations for Unerupted Teeth. *J. Biol. Regul. Homeost. Agents* **2015**, *29*, 515–520. [PubMed]
4. Betts, N.J.; Vanarsdall, R.L.; Barber, H.D.; Higgins-Barber, K.; Fonseca, R.J. Diagnosis and Treatment of Transverse Maxillary Deficiency. *Int. J. Adult Orthodon. Orthognath. Surg.* **1995**, *10*, 75–96. [PubMed]
5. Gábris, K.; Tarján, I.; Fábián, G.; Kaán, M.; Szakály, T.; Orosz, M. Frequency of supernumerary teeth and possibilities of treatment. *Fogorv. Sz.* **2001**, *94*, 53–57. [PubMed]
6. Jain, S.; Raza, M.; Sharma, P.; Kumar, P. Unraveling Impacted Maxillary Incisors: The Why, When, and How. *Int. J. Clin. Pediatr. Dent.* **2021**, *14*, 149–157. [CrossRef]
7. Brin, I.; Zilberman, Y.; Azaz, B. The Unerupted Maxillary Central Incisor: Review of Its Etiology and Treatment. *ASDC J. Dent. Child.* **1982**, *49*, 352–356.
8. Chaushu, S.; Becker, T.; Becker, A. Impacted Central Incisors: Factors Affecting Prognosis and Treatment Duration. *Am. J. Orthod. Dentofac. Orthop.* **2015**, *147*, 355–362. [CrossRef]
9. Laudadio, C.; Inchingolo, A.D.; Malcangi, G.; Limongelli, L.; Marinelli, G.; Coloccia, G.; Montenegro, V.; Patano, A.; Inchingolo, F.; Bordea, I.R.; et al. Management of Anterior Open-Bite in the Deciduous, Mixed and Permanent Dentition Stage: A Descriptive Review. *J. Biol. Regul. Homeost. Agents* **2021**, *35*, 271–281. [CrossRef]
10. Chaushu, S.; Zilberman, Y.; Becker, A. Maxillary Incisor Impaction and Its Relationship to Canine Displacement. *Am. J. Orthod. Dentofac. Orthop.* **2003**, *124*, 144–150; discussion 150. [CrossRef]
11. Inchingolo, A.D.; Patano, A.; Coloccia, G.; Ceci, S.; Inchingolo, A.M.; Marinelli, G.; Malcangi, G.; Montenegro, V.; Laudadio, C.; Palmieri, G.; et al. Genetic Pattern, Orthodontic and Surgical Management of Multiple Supplementary Impacted Teeth in a Rare, Cleidocranial Dysplasia Patient: A Case Report. *Medicina* **2021**, *57*, 1350. [CrossRef]
12. Das, D.; Misra, J. Surgical Management of Impacted Incisors in Associate with Supernumerary Teeth: A Combine Case Report of Spontaneous Eruption and Orthodontic Extrusion. *J. Indian Soc. Pedod. Prev. Dent.* **2012**, *30*, 329. [CrossRef]
13. Alsweed, A.A.; Al-sughier, Z. Surgical Management of Unerupted Permanent Maxillary Central Incisors Due to Presence of Two Supernumerary Teeth. *Int. J. Clin. Pediatr. Dent.* **2020**, *13*, 421–424. [CrossRef]
14. Zilberman, Y.; Malron, M.; Shteyer, A. Assessment of 100 Children in Jerusalem with Supernumerary Teeth in the Premaxillary Region. *ASDC J. Dent. Child.* **1992**, *59*, 44–47.
15. Rajab, L.D.; Hamdan, M.A.M. Supernumerary Teeth: Review of the Literature and a Survey of 152 Cases. *Int. J. Paediatr. Dent.* **2002**, *12*, 244–254. [CrossRef]
16. Šarac, Z.; Zovko, R.; Cvitanović, S.; Goršeta, K.; Glavina, D. Fusion of Unerupted Mesiodens with a Regular Maxillary Central Incisor: A Diagnostic and Therapeutic Challenge. *Acta Stomatol. Croat.* **2021**, *55*, 325–331. [CrossRef]
17. Marinelli, G.; Inchingolo, A.D.; Inchingolo, A.M.; Malcangi, G.; Limongelli, L.; Montenegro, V.; Coloccia, G.; Laudadio, C.; Patano, A.; Inchingolo, F.; et al. White Spot Lesions in Orthodontics: Prevention and Treatment. A Descriptive Review. *J. Biol. Regul. Homeost. Agents* **2021**, *35*, 227–240. [CrossRef]
18. Montenegro, V.; Inchingolo, A.D.; Malcangi, G.; Limongelli, L.; Marinelli, G.; Coloccia, G.; Laudadio, C.; Patano, A.; Inchingolo, F.; Bordea, I.R.; et al. Compliance of Children with Removable Functional Appliance with Microchip Integrated during Covid-19 Pandemic: A Systematic Review. *J. Biol. Regul. Homeost. Agents* **2021**, *35*, 365–377.
19. Tanki, J.Z. Impacted Maxillary Incisors: Causes, Diagnosis and Management. *IOSR-JDMS* **2013**, *5*, 41–45. [CrossRef]
20. Seehra, J.; Yaqoob, O.; Patel, S.; O'Neill, J.; Bryant, C.; Noar, J.; Morris, D.; Cobourne, M.T. National Clinical Guidelines for the Management of Unerupted Maxillary Incisors in Children. *Br. Dent. J.* **2018**, *224*, 779–785. [CrossRef]

21. Cantore, S.; Ballini, A.; Farronato, D.; Malcangi, G.; Dipalma, G.; Assandri, F.; Garagiola, U.; Inchingolo, F.; De Vito, D.; Cirulli, N. Evaluation of an Oral Appliance in Patients with Mild to Moderate Obstructive Sleep Apnea Syndrome Intolerant to Continuous Positive Airway Pressure Use: Preliminary Results. *Int. J. Immunopathol. Pharm.* **2016**, *29*, 267–273. [CrossRef]
22. Grassi, F.R.; Rapone, B.; Scarano Catanzaro, F.; Corsalini, M.; Kalemaj, Z. Effectiveness of Computer-Assisted Anesthetic Delivery System (Sta^{TM}) in Dental Implant Surgery: A Prospective Study. *Oral Implant.* **2017**, *10*, 381–389. [CrossRef]
23. Corsalini, M.; Di Venere, D.; Carossa, M.; Ripa, M.; Sportelli, P. Comparative Clinical Study between Zirconium-Ceramic and Metal-Ceramic Fixed Rehabilitations. *Oral Implantol.* **2018**, *11*, 150–160.
24. Lorusso, F.; Noumbissi, S.; Francesco, I.; Rapone, B.; Khater, A.G.A.; Scarano, A. Scientific Trends in Clinical Research on Zirconia Dental Implants: A Bibliometric Review. *Materials* **2020**, *13*, 5534. [CrossRef]
25. Pavoni, C.; Franchi, L.; Laganà, G.; Baccetti, T.; Cozza, P. Management of Impacted Incisors Following Surgery to Remove Obstacles to Eruption: A Prospective Clinical Trial. *Pediatr. Dent.* **2013**, *35*, 364–368.
26. Orthodontic Treatment of Impacted Teeth-Adrian Becker-John Wiley and Sons Ltd. | IBS. Available online: https://www.ibs.it/orthodontic-treatment-of-impacted-teeth-libro-inglese-adrian-becker/e/9781444336757 (accessed on 7 February 2022).
27. Adina, S.; Dipalma, G.; Bordea, I.R.; Lucaciu, O.; Feurdean, C.; Inchingolo, A.D.; Septimiu, R.; Malcangi, G.; Cantore, S.; Martin, D.; et al. Orthopedic Joint Stability Influences Growth and Maxillary Development: Clinical Aspects. *J. Biol. Regul. Homeost. Agents* **2020**, *34*, 747–756. [CrossRef]
28. Di Venere, D.; Nardi, G.M.; Lacarbonara, V.; Laforgia, A.; Stefanachi, G.; Corsalini, M.; Grassi, F.R.; Rapone, B.; Pettini, F. Early Mandibular Canine-Lateral Incisor Transposition: Case Report. *Oral Implant.* **2017**, *10*, 181–189. [CrossRef]
29. Coloccia, G.; Inchingolo, A.D.; Inchingolo, A.M.; Malcangi, G.; Montenegro, V.; Patano, A.; Marinelli, G.; Laudadio, C.; Limongelli, L.; Di Venere, D.; et al. Effectiveness of Dental and Maxillary Transverse Changes in Tooth-Borne, Bone-Borne, and Hybrid Palatal Expansion through Cone-Beam Tomography: A Systematic Review of the Literature. *Medicina* **2021**, *57*, 288. [CrossRef] [PubMed]
30. Cardarelli, D.F. Il trattamento funzionale elastodontico con apparecchi AMCOP: Funzione, estetica e postura. *Dental Tribune*, 3 July 2019.
31. Özer, M.; Şener, I.; Bayram, M. Bilaterally Impacted Maxillary Central Incisors: Surgical Exposure and Orthodontic Treatment: A Case Report. *J. Contemp. Dent. Pract.* **2006**, *7*, 98–105. [CrossRef]
32. Farronato, M.; Farronato, D.; Inchingolo, F.; Grassi, L.; Lanteri, V.; Maspero, C. Evaluation of Dental Surface after De-Bonding Orthodontic Bracket Bonded with a Novel Fluorescent Composite: In Vitro Comparative Study. *Appl. Sci.* **2021**, *11*, 6354. [CrossRef]
33. Becker, A.; Brin, I.; Ben-Bassat, Y.; Zilberman, Y.; Chaushu, S. Closed-Eruption Surgical Technique for Impacted Maxillary Incisors: A Postorthodontic Periodontal Evaluation. *Am. J. Orthod. Dentofac. Orthop.* **2002**, *122*, 9–14. [CrossRef]
34. Inchingolo, A.D.; Patano, A.; Coloccia, G.; Ceci, S.; Inchingolo, A.M.; Marinelli, G.; Malcangi, G.; Montenegro, V.; Laudadio, C.; Pede, C.D.; et al. The Efficacy of a New AMCOP®Elastodontic Protocol for Orthodontic Interceptive Treatment: A Case Series and Literature Overview. *Int. J. Environ. Res. Public Health* **2022**, *19*, 988. [CrossRef]
35. Tsai, T.-P. Surgical Repositioning of an Impacted Dilacerated Incisor in Mixed Dentition. *J. Am. Dent. Assoc.* **2002**, *133*, 61–66. [CrossRef]
36. Farronato, G.; Giannini, L.; Galbiati, G.; Maspero, C. A 5-Year Longitudinal Study of Survival Rate and Periodontal Parameter Changes at Sites of Dilacerated Maxillary Central Incisors. *Prog. Orthod.* **2014**, *15*, 3. [CrossRef]
37. Patianna, A.G.; Ballini, A.; Meneghello, M.; Cantore, S.; Inchingolo, A.M.; Dipalma, G.; Inchingolo, A.D.; Inchingolo, F.; Malcangi, G.; Lucchese, A.; et al. Comparison of Conventional Orthognathic Surgery and "Surgery-First" Protocol: A New Weapon against Time. *J. Biol. Regul. Homeost. Agents* **2019**, *33*, 59–67, DENTAL SUPPLEMENT.
38. Ho, K.; Liao, Y. Predictors of Surgical-Orthodontic Treatment Duration of Unilateral Impacted Maxillary Central Incisors. *Orthod. Craniofacial Res.* **2011**, *14*, 175–180. [CrossRef]
39. Maspero, C.; Cappella, A.; Dolci, C.; Cagetti, M.G.; Inchingolo, F.; Sforza, C. Is Orthodontic Treatment with Microperforations Worth It? A Scoping Review. *Children* **2022**, *9*, 208. [CrossRef]
40. Corsalini, M.; Di Venere, D.; Sportelli, P.; Magazzino, D.; Ripa, M.; Cantatore, F.; Cagnetta, C.; Rinaldis, C.; Montemurro, N.; Giacomo, et al. Evaluation of Prosthetic Quality and Masticatory Efficiency in Patients with Total Removable Prosthesis Study of 12 Cases. *ORAL Implantol.* **2018**, *11*, 230–240.
41. Chew, M.T.; Ong, M.M.-A. Orthodontic-Surgical Management of an Impacted Dilacerated Maxillary Central Incisor: A Clinical Case Report. *Pediatr. Dent.* **2004**, *26*, 341–344.
42. Vermette, M.E.; Kokich, V.G.; Kennedy, D.B. Uncovering Labially Impacted Teeth: Apically Positioned Flap and Closed-Eruption Techniques. *Angle Orthod.* **1995**, *65*, 23–32. [CrossRef]
43. Quaglia, E.; Moscufo, L.; Corsalini, M.; Coscia, D.; Sportelli, P.; Cantatore, F.; Rinaldis, C.; Rapone, B.; Carossa, M.; Carossa, S. Polyamide vs Silk Su.utures in the Healing of Postextraction Sockets: A Split Mouth Study. *ORAL Implantol.* **2018**, *11*, 115–120. [CrossRef]
44. Rapone, B.; Ferrara, E.; Corsalini, M.; Converti, I.; Grassi, F.R.; Santacroce, L.; Topi, S.; Gnoni, A.; Scacco, S.; Scarano, A.; et al. The Effect of Gaseous Ozone Therapy in Conjunction with Periodontal Treatment on Glycated Hemoglobin Level in Subjects with Type 2 Diabetes Mellitus: An Unmasked Randomized Controlled Trial. *Int. J. Environ. Res. Public Health* **2020**, *17*, E5467. [CrossRef]

45. Grassi, F.R.; Grassi, R.; Rapone, B.; Alemanno, G.; Balena, A.; Kalemaj, Z. Dimensional Changes of Buccal Bone Plate in Immediate Implants Inserted through Open Flap, Open Flap and Bone Grafting and Flapless Techniques: A Cone-Beam Computed Tomography Randomized Controlled Clinical Trial. *Clin. Oral Implant. Res.* **2019**, *30*, 1155–1164. [CrossRef]
46. Rapone, B.; Corsalini, M.; Converti, I.; Loverro, M.T.; Gnoni, A.; Trerotoli, P.; Ferrara, E. Does Periodontal Inflammation Affect Type 1 Diabetes in Childhood and Adolescence? A Meta-Analysis. *Front. Endocrinol.* **2020**, *11*, 278. [CrossRef]
47. Rapone, B.; Ferrara, E.; Santacroce, L.; Cesarano, F.; Arazzi, M.; Liberato, L.D.; Scacco, S.; Grassi, R.; Grassi, F.R.; Gnoni, A.; et al. Periodontal Microbiological Status Influences the Occurrence of Cyclosporine-A and Tacrolimus-Induced Gingival Overgrowth. *Antibiotics* **2019**, *8*, 124. [CrossRef]
48. Patano, A.; Cirulli, N.; Beretta, M.; Plantamura, P.; Inchingolo, A.D.; Inchingolo, A.M.; Bordea, I.R.; Malcangi, G.; Marinelli, G.; Scarano, A.; et al. Education Technology in Orthodontics and Paediatric Dentistry during the COVID-19 Pandemic: A Systematic Review. *Int. J. Environ. Res. Public Health* **2021**, *18*, 6046. [CrossRef]
49. Cantore, S.; Ballini, A.; De Vito, D.; Martelli, F.S.; Georgakopoulos, I.; Almasri, M.; Dibello, V.; Altini, V.; Farronato, G.; Dipalma, G.; et al. Characterization of Human Apical Papilla-Derived Stem Cells. *J. Biol. Regul. Homeost. Agents* **2017**, *31*, 901–910.
50. Ballini, A.; Cantore, S.; Fotopoulou, E.A.; Georgakopoulos, I.P.; Athanasiou, E.; Bellos, D.; Paduanelli, G.; Saini, R.; Dipalma, G.; Inchingolo, F. Combined Sea Salt-Based Oral Rinse with Xylitol in Orthodontic Patients: Clinical and Microbiological Study. *J. Biol. Regul. Homeost. Agents* **2019**, *33*, 263–268.
51. Di Venere, D.; Pettini, F.; Nardi, G.M.; Laforgia, A.; Stefanachi, G.; Notaro, V.; Rapone, B.; Grassi, F.R.; Corsalini, M. Correlation between Parodontal Indexes and Orthodontic Retainers: Prospective Study in a Group of 16 Patients. *Oral Implantol.* **2017**, *10*, 78. [CrossRef]

MDPI
St. Alban-Anlage 66
4052 Basel
Switzerland
Tel. +41 61 683 77 34
Fax +41 61 302 89 18
www.mdpi.com

Applied Sciences Editorial Office
E-mail: applsci@mdpi.com
www.mdpi.com/journal/applsci

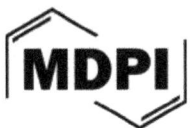

www.ingramcontent.com/pod-product-compliance
Lightning Source LLC
LaVergne TN
LVHW070541100526
838202LV00012B/337